ECG Acquisition and Automated Remote Processing

Rajarshi Gupta · Madhuchhanda Mitra
Jitendranath Bera

ECG Acquisition and Automated Remote Processing

Springer

Rajarshi Gupta
Madhuchhanda Mitra
Jitendranath Bera
Department of Applied Physics
University of Calcutta
Kolkata, West Bengal
India

ISBN 978-81-322-1556-1 ISBN 978-81-322-1557-8 (eBook)
DOI 10.1007/978-81-322-1557-8
Springer New Delhi Heidelberg New York Dordrecht London

Library of Congress Control Number: 2013942977

Printed on acid-free paper

Springer is part of Springer Science+Business Media (www.springer.com)

Foreword

I am glad to note that a monograph entitled "ECG Acquisition and Automated Remote Processing," is published by M/s. Springer India. This is really a very timely and state-of-the-art publication in the area of Biomedical Instrumentation. The authors of this monograph are a group of dedicated faculty members attached to the "Biomedical Signal Acquisition and Processing" unit in the Department of Applied Physics, University of Calcutta.

If the twentieth century has seen spectacular advances in the area of Physical Sciences, then the twenty-first century is going to be dominated by the Biological Sciences. One of the very important focal areas in the Biological Sciences must be related to Healthcare and Medical Science. As a consequence, a new multidisciplinary area of study has emerged, as Biomedical Engineering.

Modern day Biological Science and Engineering has been highly dependent on developments in Physics and Electrical Engineering, as has been found during the last few decades. The advances in Electron Microscopy, Nuclear Magnetic Resonance, Tomography, Laser Technology, Control Engineering, Solid State Electronics, Computer Technology, Sensor Technology, Signal processing, and Image processing are some of the areas that have immensely helped Biomedical Researchers from both the therapeutic and diagnostic points of view.

Heart, being a vital and complex organ of the human body, needs special attention for its monitoring. A very useful noninvasive technique to monitor the activity of the heart system is to study the ECG signals and get analytical information about its functioning.

This monograph is dedicated to the acquisition, analysis, and transmission of electrical signals generated by the activities of the cardiovascular organ. ECG signals need complex analysis to extract useful information about the health of the heart. Although for a pretty long time, it is being attempted to gather this information for diagnostic purposes, shortcomings in the analytical tools create some problems. This is why this topic has attracted the attention of researchers, world over, who are equipped with such modern analytical tools to attack this problem.

In this monograph there are six chapters and at the end of each individual chapter there are references, which give the future workers scope for study in this field.

Students at the undergraduate and postgraduate levels in Biomedical Engineering and Biomedical Instrumentation will find this monograph very useful for their coursework. I must thank the authors for their endeavor.

Kolkata, India, May 19, 2013

Prof. Dr. Dilip Kumar Basu
Former Vice Chancellor, Burdwan University
Bardhaman, West Bengal
India

Former Vice Chancellor, Tripura University
Agartala
India

Preface

Healthcare has been identified as one of the emerging areas of research in the current century. In spite of the remarkable development of science and technology in the last four decades, the average mortality rates have increased in most countries. Cardiovascular Diseases (CVD) remain as the dominant killer all over the world. As per statistics from World Health Organization (WHO), an estimated 17.3 million people died from CVD in 2008, representing 30% of all global deaths. Of these deaths, an estimated 7.3 million were due to coronary heart disease and 6.2 million were due to stroke. It is predicted that by the year 2030, 23.6 million people will die from CVDs, and the worst affected region will be SouthEast Asia. Medical science has achieved significant progress in the recent years, mainly contributed by research from bioinformatics, molecular biology, genetics, nanotechnology, drug research, and peripheral sciences. As a result, human civilization has been able to overpower many incurable diseases. At the same time, newer and complex forms of diseases have come out and put tougher challenges before the medical scientists.

The marriage between medical science and technology has given birth to a new discipline, named biomedical engineering, which is contributed by some core and multidisciplinary engineering disciplines like Electrical, Electronics and Communication, Instrumentation, Mechanical, and VLSI. Technologists have developed diagnostics tools and devices to extract pathological information from patients and present them in a suitable format as an aid to the medical expert to support his therapeutic actions. Electrocardiogram (ECG), the small potentials generated by the heart muscles, is perhaps the most explored medical signal by the biomedical research community, due to its importance in overall healthiness of a human being. Invention of the ECG machine by Willem Einthoven in the early twentieth century is considered as one of the pioneering landmarks in the history of biomedical science. After that, various types of biomedical equipments and devices have been developed which are capable of providing a very high degree of accuracy. A major impetus to this was development of imaging equipments like ultrasonograph, computed tomography, etc., which are completely noninvasive in nature.

Poor doctor to patient ratio is one of the persistent problem in the underdeveloped and developing nations. Due to various socio-economic factors and lack of proper healthcare policies, the number of qualified medical professionals for catering the need of rural patients is inadequate. A remedial measure toward this problem was introduction of telehealth services, where the physician is supplied with the medical signals from a remote patient using various communication technologies. In advanced nations, this remote healthcare service is now a standard practice extended to the remotest primary clinics in rural areas. However, in developing nations this facility is not so widespread in regular service. Development of smart, powerful, miniature devices is still an active area of research with the objective of easy acquisition, fast processing, and seamless communication of medical data to the remote end physician. In the context of developing nations like India, easy operability and affordability are the key driving factors which should drive the technology for delivering healthcare service to the general population. Many Indian institutions are engaged in this area of research.

This monograph is a small and humble contribution from the Biomedical Signal Acquisition and Processing Research Group at Department of Applied Physics, University of Calcutta, India. This book is written with the outcome of some experimental developments of a prototype telecardiology system. The book is addressed to a broad audience. It is expected to be useful to undergraduate and postgraduate students of Biomedical Engineering, Electrical Engineering, Instrumentation Engineering, and researchers working in the similar area. One advantageous feature for the readers is that all the algorithm outlines are presented at the end of chapter appendix, so that new researchers can develop or customize their own applications. A brief review of the main focal subjects is provided in the respective chapters. The publications from our research group relevant to the topic are indicated at the end of each chapter. This book is only meant to create interest and initiate more work among the researchers and carry the concept further. Some pictures, tables, and illustrations are reproduced from earlier publications and the copyrights will rest with the original publishers.

The authors welcome comments and suggestions from the readers.

Kolkata, India

Rajarshi Gupta
Madhuchhanda Mitra
Jitendranath Bera

Acknowledgments

The authors are thankful to the faculty members and staff of Department of Applied Physics, University of Calcutta for the support and cooperation. The experiments, a few results of which are shown in some chapters, are supported by equipments purchased from Technical Education Quality Improvement Programme (TEQIP) Phase-I at UCT, CU. Our research group received support from SAP DRS-I programme from University Grants Commission (UGC) and FIST project from Department of Science and Technology (DST), Government of India. A special mention of Prof. Samarjit Sengupta, former Head, Department of Applied Physics for his advice, encouragement, and close association with our research group. The authors extend their thanks to Prof. Dilip Kumar Basu, former Vice Chancellor, Tripura University, India for writing the Foreword of this book. The authors express their sincere gratitude to Springer India for publication of this book.

The authors also acknowledge the support received from their family members.

Rajarshi Gupta
Madhuchhanda Mitra
Jitendranath Bera

Contents

Acronyms

AV Node	Atrioventricular node
ATA	American Telemedicine Association
AHA	American Heart Association
ANSI	American National Standards Institute
AAMI	Association for the Advancement of Medical Instrumentation
ASK	Amplitude shift keying
ARQ	Automatic repeat request
AZTEC	Amplitude zonal time epoch coding
ANN	Artificial neural network
BEC	Burst error correction
BPSK	Binary phase shift keying
BP	Blood pressure
BER	Bit error rate
BW	Baseline wander
BPM	Bi-phase modulation
CRO	Cathode ray oscilloscope
CR	Compression ratio
CSE	Common standard of electrocardiogram
CMRR	Common mode rejection ratio
CORTES	Coordinate reduction time encoding system
DSP	Digital signal processing
DCT	Discrete cosine transform
DFT	Discrete fourier transform
DWT	Discrete wavelet transform
DAS	Data acquisition system
DDC	Direct data compression
DSSS	Direct sequence spread spectrum
EMD	Empirical mode decomposition
ECG	Electrocardiogram
EMG	Electromyogram
EIA	Electronics Industries Association
EPABX	Electronic private automatic branch exchange
FP	False positive

FDA	Food and Drug Administration
FCC	Federal Communication Commission
FSK	Frequency shift keying
FDM	Frequency division multiplexing
GSM	Global system of mobiles
HEMA	Health Industry Manufacturers Association
HT	Hilbert transform
HTML	Hyper text markup language
IMRR	Isolation mode rejection ratio
INA	Instrumentation amplifier
ISI	Inter symbol interference
ITC	Information and Communication Technology
ICA	Independent component analysis
ISDN	Integrated services digital network
IEC	International Electrotechnical Commission
KLT	Karhumen Loève transform
MAE	Maximum absolute error
MCU	Microcontroller unit
MI	Myocardial infarction
MSC	Mobile satellite communication
MSE	Mean square error
MLP	Multilayer perceptron
NRF	Noise reduction factors
OFDM	Orthogonal frequency division multiplexing
OSI	Open system interface
OOK	Orthogonal frequency-division multiplexing
PDA	Personal digital assistant
PE	Packet error
PRD	Percentage root mean squared difference
PNR	Percentage noise retention ratio
PSK	Phase shift keying
NRFIR	Non recursive finite impulse response
PVE	Peak value extractor
PSTN	Public switched telephone network
PLI	Power line interference
PVC	Premature ventricular contraction
PCA	Principal component analysis
QPSK	Quadrature phase shift keying
QS	Quality score
SNR	Signal to noise ratio
SA Node	Sinoatrial node
SAPA	Scan along polynomial approximation
SCP	Standard communication protocol
TP	Turning point
TIA	Telecommunications Industry Association

TDM	Time division multiplexing
TP	True positive
TCP/IP	Transmission control protocol/Internet protocol
TN	True negative
UART	Universal asynchronous receiver transmitter
WCT	Wilson central terminal

Chapter 1
Introduction

1.1 Introduction

Even more than a century after its invention, electrocardiogram (ECG) still remains the primary choice of the physicians for preliminary level investigation of patients against chest pains and a helpful clue to the generalized disorders that affect the rest of the body too. It is a simple non-invasive technique to explore the cardiac functions of a patient. This chapter is aimed to discuss the basics of ECG, its genesis, and lead systems. This is followed by a discussion on current health-care scenario and context of introducing telehealth facility and its significance in the developing nations.

1.2 Heart and Cardiovascular System

Human heart is a four-chambered, hollow, and flexible organ that collects impure blood from the other organs, purifies it, and then circulates oxygenated blood to the whole body. It is placed in the thoracic chamber, anterior to the vertebral column and posterior to the sternum, slightly offset to the left. Depending on the age, it weights between 250 and 350 g. Human heart consists of two pairs of atria and ventricles, longitudinally connected. The heart along with the network of veins (carry deoxygenated blood) and arteries (carry oxygenated blood) forms the cardiovascular system to supply blood to the whole body. The word cardiac is derived from Greek word 'kardia,' meaning 'related to the heart.' Considering its importance to support life, heart is considered as one of the three most important body organs, along with kidney and central nervous system. The heart is cushioned in a two-layered sac called pericardium. The outer layer, named fibrous pericardium, protects the heart against mechanical damage and prevents its overfilling with blood. The outer wall of the heart consists of three layers, viz. epicardium, myocardium, and endocardium. The first one forms the inner layer of pericardium, and the last one forms the heart chambers. Between the heart chambers and outlet

R. Gupta et al., *ECG Acquisition and Automated Remote Processing*,
DOI: 10.1007/978-81-322-1557-8_1, © Springer India 2014

from ventricles, unidirectional flow of blood is controlled by two types of valves, viz. tricuspid valve and mitral valve. There is a thick wall of muscle, named septum, which separates the right side and the left side of the heart. More details of human heart physiology can be found at [1, 2].

The atria receive the blood from the body, and ventricles supply the blood. The pair of atria and ventricles work in tandem, i.e., they contract and expand together to collect and supply blood, respectively. In between these two operations, there is an important function of purification, which is performed by sending the impure (deoxygenated) blood to the lungs. To achieve this, the right ventricle sends the impure blood to the lungs and receives the pure blood at the left atria.

A complete cardiac cycle consists of collection of blood from body organs, its purification, and sending it back to the whole body. Figures 1.1 and 1.2 describe the schematic circulatory flow of blood between heart chambers and body organs for one cycle. Deoxygenated blood from the upper and lower parts of the body is brought through superior vena cava and inferior vena cava, respectively, to the right atrium to force fill it. When the pressure inside the right atria reaches a certain value, the tricuspid valve opens to give the passage for blood to the right ventricle. When the right ventricle is filled up, the pulmonary valve opens to pump the blood to the lungs through pulmonary artery. In the lungs, the purification (oxygenation) of the blood takes place by transfer of O_2 and CO_2 by their difference of partial pressure between inside and outside of alveolar sacs. The purified blood is brought back to the left ventricle by pulmonary vein to force fill it, till the pressure reached a certain value, when the bicuspid valve (also called mitral valve) opens. The ventricle receives the oxygenated blood and then finally pumps it to the whole body through the aortic semilunar valve to the aorta. The

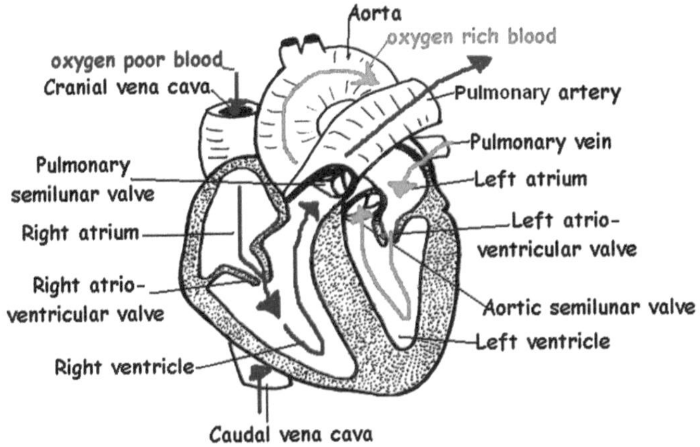

Fig. 1.1 Circulatory blood flow through the heart chambers

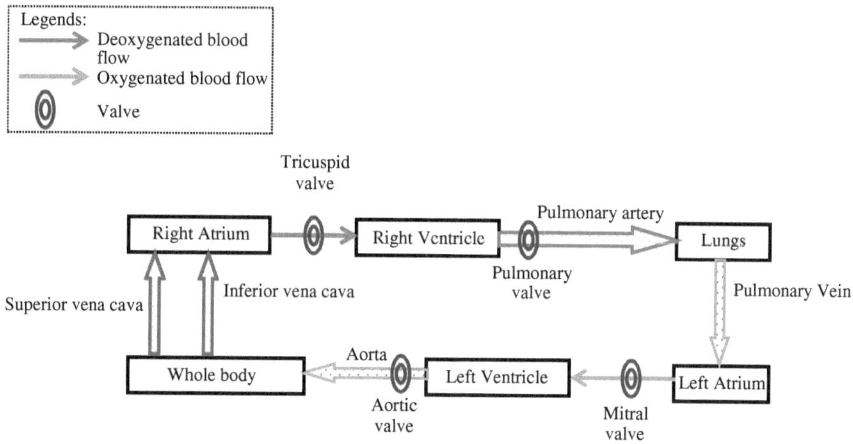

Fig. 1.2 Schematic blood flow direction between heart chambers

delivered blood is divided into major arteries which supply them to the lower and upper parts of the body to feed each body cell. The pumping action of the heart supports the following circulatory systems:

Pulmonary circulation: This supports blood circulation to the lungs for purification.
Systemic circulation: This supports blood circulation to the entire body except the lungs.
Coronary circulation: To function properly, the heart cells need oxygenated blood. Coronary circulation takes care of this.

A healthy adult human heart contracts (or expands) 72–80 times per minute. Since the pumping action required for systemic circulation is much greater than pulmonary circulation, the left atrium and left ventricle are more muscular than right counterparts.

1.3 Genesis of the Electrocardiogram

The mechanical action of the heart is due to generation of small electrical impulses and their propagation on the heart surface. ECG represents time-averaged representation of these electrical potentials picked up by placing electrodes on body surface. As a convention, an activity is recorded as positive (negative) when the resulting electrical impulses move toward (away from) the electrode.

The electrical activity of heart muscles is initiated at sinoatrial (SA) node located at the upper region of the right atrium. A specialized group of cells named pacemaker cells at this node spontaneously depolarize and repolarize at a rate of 60–100 times/min. The electrical impulses gradually spread over the atria at a speed of 4 m/s, causing them to contract together. This produces a noticeable deflection on the ECG record, which is named as P wave. After flowing through the atria, the electrical impulses reach at the atrioventricular (AV) node, located at the lower end of the right atria. Here, the conduction is delayed, at speed of 0.1 m/s. AV node is the only route through which these electrical impulses can reach the ventricles, since the rest of atrial myocardium is separated from the ventricles by a non-conducting ring of fibrous tissue. The conduction at the AV node provides a gap between the atrial conduction and ventricular conduction and reflected as an equipotential line, named PR segment in the ECG record. From the AV node, the electrical impulses enter the bundle of His which is bifurcated to left bundle and right bundle branches. As the impulses flow through the bundle branches, the contraction (depolarization) of the ventricles starts together. This generates a combination of sharp downward and upward deflection in the ECG record, named as QRS complex. The right bundle branch conducts the pathway of conduction to the right ventricle, while the left bundle branch is divided into anterior and posterior fascicles that conduct the wave to the left ventricle. The conduction is gradually distributed in Purkinje fibers, which are spread out to the left and right atria. Since the systemic circulation dominates in overall contraction of the ventricles in terms of muscle activity, the QRS complex mainly represents ventricular contraction due to left ventricle. During ventricular contraction, the atria also expand (repolarizes). However, the generated electrical activity due to this is very feeble and suppressed by the ventricular activity. There is a small time gap between the ventricular contraction and expansion, where no electrical activity is recorded in the ECG record. This is represented by the equipotential ST segment, after which the ventricles start expanding (repolarization) together. The ventricular repolarization is represented by a T wave in the ECG record. In certain electrodes, a U wave is recorded as small after-potentials after the T wave, representing slow repolarization of inter-ventricular septum or slow repolarization of ventricles. The cardiac events and corresponding ECG waves are summarized in Table 1.1 and Fig. 1.3.

Table 1.1 ECG waves and events

Wave/segment	Event name
P wave	Atrial depolarization
PR interval	Start of atrial depolarization to start of ventricular depolarization
QRS complex	Ventricular depolarization
ST segment	Pause in ventricular electrical activity before repolarization
T wave	Ventricular repolarization
U wave (uncertain)	Slow ventricular repolarization Or, inter-ventricular septal repolarization

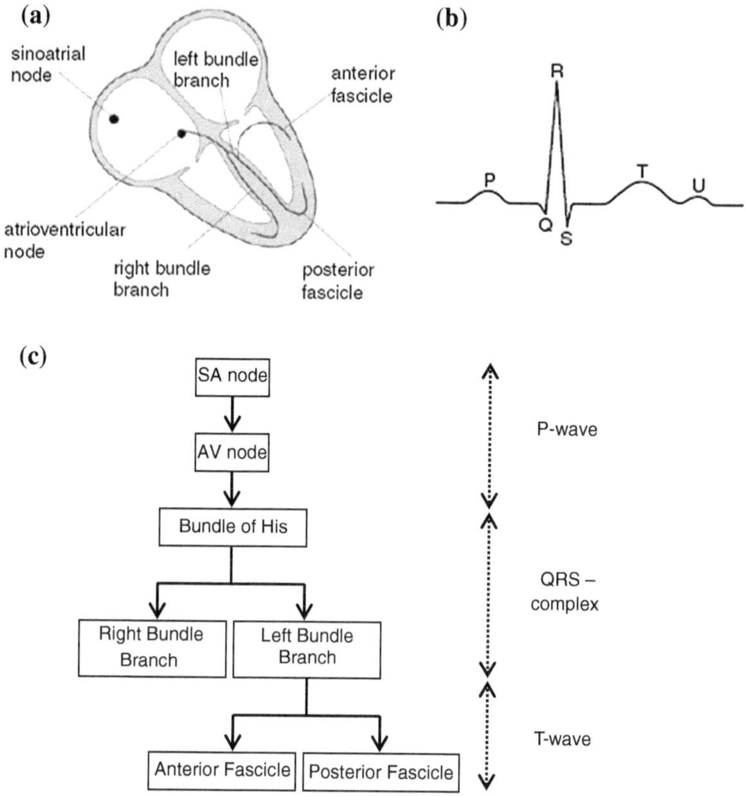

Fig. 1.3 Electrical conduction system through heart schematic. **a** Electrical conducting system of heart. **b** ECG wave. **c** Conduction pathway sequence

1.4 ECG Clinical Signatures

A complete cardiac cycle is represented by P–QRS–T waves, connected by some equipotential segments in a typical ECG wave, called a 'beat.' Most of the diagnostic information is contained in the morphology and wave duration and intervals of constituent waves. For ECG interpretations, some conventions are used for the wave durations and intervals, defined as follows:

Onset: the start or initiation of an electrical activity (repolarization or depolarization).
Offset: the end or termination of an electrical activity (repolarization or depolarization).
Wave duration (or width): time gap between the onset and offset of the same wave.
Interval: onset of one wave and offset of the other wave (or next wave).
Segment: offset of one wave and onset of the following wave.

For QRS complex, the starting is indicated by Q-onset and termination by S-offset. Most of the practical ECG records contain some baseline modulation, which appears as slow undulations of the equipotential segments PR, ST, and TP. Some researchers consider the baseline voltage in the PQ segment [3], i.e., between the P-offset and Q-onset points. However, for some abnormal ECGs, a distinct PQ segment is either not available or inclined, which poses difficulty for baseline detection. In such cases, the average amplitude of the TP segment, which is often the longest equipotential segment in an ECG wave, is taken as the baseline voltage. However, for accurate measurement on beat-to-beat basis, wave amplitudes or heights are measured with respect to a local baseline, which is obtained by averaging the amplitudes of onset and offset points of the corresponding wave. Often the clinicians define a J-point at the knee region of the ST segment as the electrical neutral voltage, which represents the electrical activity exactly between the ventricular depolarization and repolarization. However, wide variations in ST segments in diseased heart may create problem in finding the exact location of J-point in some records. Figure 1.4 shows the useful ECG features and wave durations commonly used for clinical diagnosis.

Among the common clinical signatures, distance between two consecutive *R* peaks, named RR-duration, signify heart rhythms and is used for heart rate computation. The ventricular activity (depolarization and repolarization) is recorded in the QT segment, which is the region of interest to the cardiologists for diagnosis of major cardiac diseases. Since the heart rate of a normal patient may change during continuous recording, a corrected QT interval named $(QT)_c$ is sometimes used to compensate the heart rate variation, given by Bazett's formula:

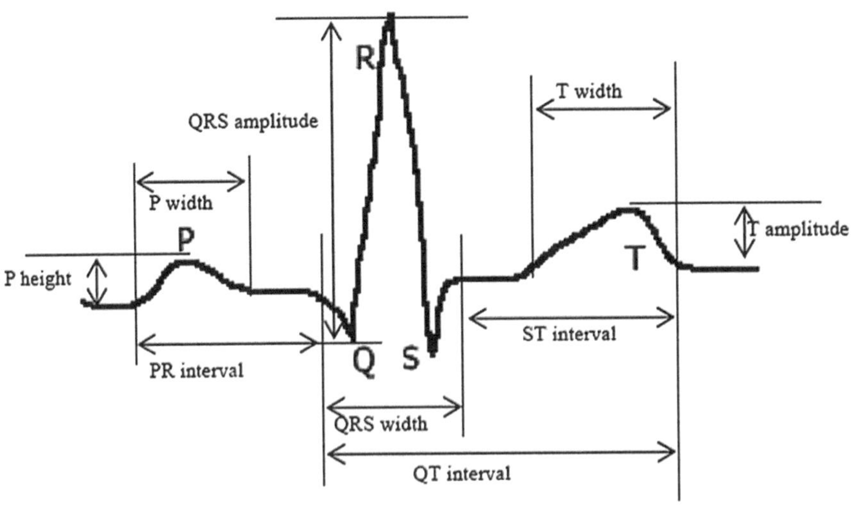

Fig. 1.4 Useful clinical signatures of ECG

Table 1.2 Common ECG signatures for clinical use

Clinical signature	Typical values (unit)	Nominal limits (unit)
P width	110 ms	±20 ms
T width	180 ms	±40 ms
PR interval	120 ms	±20 ms
QRS width	100 ms	±20 ms
QT_c interval	400 ms	±40 ms
P amplitude	0.15 mV	±005 mV
T amplitude	0.3 mV	±0.2 mV
QRS amplitude	1.2 mV	±0.5 mV

$$(\mathrm{QT})_c = \frac{\mathrm{QT\,interval}}{\sqrt{R - R\,\mathrm{duration}}} \tag{1.1}$$

Or Fridericia's formula:

$$(\mathrm{QT})_c = \frac{\mathrm{QT\,interval}}{\sqrt[3]{R - R\,\mathrm{interval}}} \tag{1.2}$$

For clinical diagnosis, the medical experts have identified some quantitative and some qualitative signatures. Some of the common clinical signatures expressed in quantitative manner are given in Table 1.2 against their nominal range for a healthy adult. However, for complete feature extraction, as many as 18 clinical signatures are reported in the literature. Some qualitative signatures used for diagnosis are inverted P wave, pathological Q wave, ST segment elevation, etc. Clinical interpretations of ECG signatures are available in [4].

Malfunctions in heart alter the clinical signatures in some way, and the medical experts assess these deviations from their nominal range to classify the patient in one or more classes. However, the actual clinical diagnosis procedure is much more complex, since many other parameters like age, sex, hereditary symptoms, food habits, and demographic factors are also taken into consideration, in addition to the fact that different diseases appear in different lead(s).

1.5 ECG Lead System

ECG lead system describes internationally accepted standards for placing electrodes on external body surface to pick up ECG signal. This provides a framework for easy reproducibility, comparison, and nomenclatures for the medical and research fraternity to describe, analyze, and interpret ECG records. The first work on ECG lead standardization was performed by W. Einthoven, who received Nobel Prize in Medicine for his work in the year 1924. Einthoven postulated that human body is a perfect sphere with homogeneous density, with the human heart located at the center. He considered three leads placed on the right arm, left arm

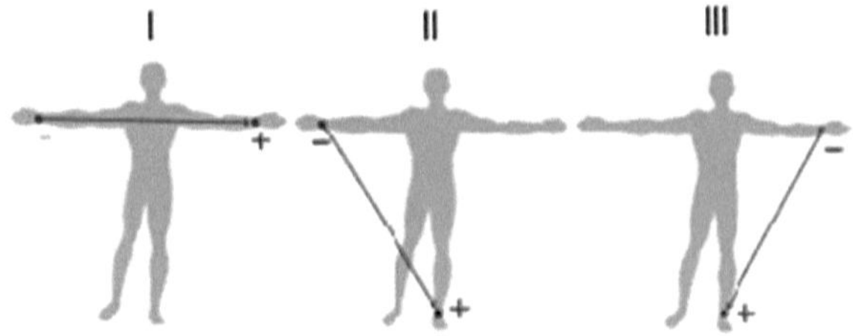

Fig. 1.5 Standard lead positions of Einthoven

and left leg of a person standing with laterally stretched hands, which forms an equilateral triangle with the vertices on a circle. Einthoven's bipolar leads, also called standard leads, are defined as

$$\text{Lead I} = V_{LA} - V_{RA} \tag{1.3}$$

$$\text{Lead II} = V_{LL} - V_{RA} \tag{1.4}$$

$$\text{Lead III} = V_{LL} - V_{LA} \tag{1.5}$$

where

V_{LA} : potential of the left arm.
V_{RA}: potential of the right arm.
V_{LL}: potential of the left leg.

The lead positions and connections for the standard leads or limb leads developed by Einthoven are shown in Fig. 1.5.

Later on, Frank Wilson defined and standardized unipolar leads with three unipolar limb leads and six precordial chest leads, measured w.r.t. a reference terminal outside the body, named Wilson central terminal (WCT). WCT is realized as a resistive network using 5-kΩ resistances and given as

$$V_{WCT} = \frac{1}{3}(V_{LA} + V_{RA} + V_{LL}) \tag{1.6}$$

The precordial chest leads are defined as

$$\text{Lead VL} = V_{LA} - V_{WCT} \tag{1.7}$$

$$\text{Lead VR} = V_{RA} - V_{WCT} \tag{1.8}$$

$$\text{Lead VF} = V_{LL} - V_{WCT} \tag{1.9}$$

Later on, E. Goldberger modified the precordial leads to develop 'Augmented Limb Leads,' aVR, aVL, and aVF, respectively, by opening the exploring lead connections with the WCT. The lead connections are given in Fig. 1.6. The lead positions are given in Table 1.1.

The chest leads *v*1, *v*2, *v*3, *v*4, *v*5, and *v*6 measure the cardiac potentials at specified intercostal spaces of the chest w.r.t. WCT. These six leads define the

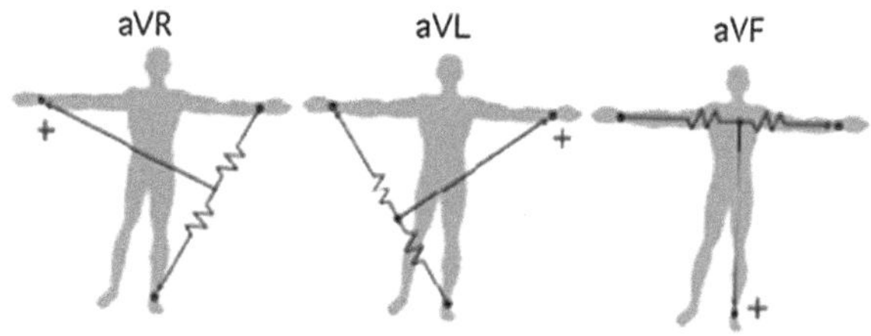

Fig. 1.6 Augmented lead positions and connections

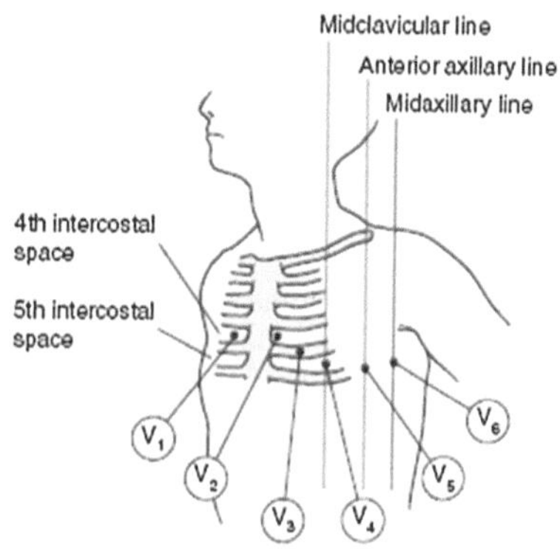

Fig. 1.7 Precordial lead positions

Table 1.3 Lead positions of precordial or chest leads

Lead name	Position
V1	Right 4th intercostal space
V2	Left 4th intercostal space
V3	Halfway between v2 and v4
V4	Left 5th intercostal space
V5	Horizontal to v4, anterior auxiliary plane
V6	Horizontal to v5, mid-auxiliary plane

ECG in a horizontal plane. The lead positions are shown in Fig. 1.7 and Table 1.3. The six frontal plane leads (I, II, III) and six horizontal plane leads constitute 12-lead ECG system which is by far the most common and accepted method of mapping of ECG signal from a patient. More details of ECG lead systems can be found at [5].

1.6 ECG Recording

ECG record in a clinical set up is generated through an electrocardiograph machine, with electrodes connected to the patient body. It incorporates an amplifier, filter, patient isolation, and mechanical printing arrangement. A thermally sensitive, graduated strip chart paper is driven at a speed of 25 mm/s (most recommended), and it generates the impression by a moving stylus controlled by amplifier output. Each smallest square on the paper record along x-axis (time) represents 40 ms, and same along y-axis (millivolt amplitudes) represents 0.1 mV. A physician can calculate the wave amplitudes, durations, and intervals from the graduations very easily. Old or traditional recordings facilitate sequential recording, i.e., one lead plot can be obtained at a time by mechanical switching arrangement. However, most modern electrocardiograph machines are enabled with direct computer interface and allow simultaneous, multilead recording.

1.7 Evolution and Practice of Telemedicine and Telecardiology

Biotelemetry is the common technique which involves collection of physiological data at one place and its transmission to another place using a suitable communication media for recording, interpretation, and analysis [6, 7]. In clinical practice, however, the term 'telemedicine' [8] is more frequently used. Telemedicine is the integrated technology platform where a remote patient can be examined and monitored through a communication link by a remote physician. American Telemedicine Association (ATA) [9], one of the leading professional organization advocating the use of remote diagnostics to improve quality, equity, and affordability of health care throughout the world, defines the telemedicine as, "Telemedicine is the use of medical information exchanged from one site to another via electronic communications to improve patients' health status. Closely associated with telemedicine is the term 'telehealth,' which is often used to encompass a broader definition of remote health care that does not always involve clinical services. Videoconferencing, transmission of still images, e-health including patient portals, remote monitoring of vital signs, continuing medical education and nursing call centers are all considered part of telemedicine and telehealth". Use of information and communication technology (ICT) for health-care service is well established in advanced nations, where the basic health and supporting infrastructure are adequate to deliver a quality health-care service to the common people. However, in most of the developing nations like India, the patient-to-doctor ratio is very high. The advanced health-care facilities are city centric. The following reasons can be identified as the principal causes for promotion of telehealth services in developing nations:

1. Disparity in health-care service distribution among rural and urban areas.
2. Poor rural health-care infrastructure.
3. Inadequate number of medical practitioners and paramedics in rural health-care centers.
4. Poor road connectivity of city-based hospitals with remote districts.
5. Tendency of city-based medical specialists to practice their profession around densely populated city areas.
6. Poor doctor-to-patient ratio.

Some references are obtained from published articles regarding the aforementioned causes. In [10], a detailed statistics is provided for the opportunities and scope of improvement of telemedicine services in India. It mentions that around 80% of the main health-care centers are based on cities, which host only 30% of the total population. Doctor-to-patient ratio in India is typically 60 per lakh, compared to 250+ per lakh in advanced countries [11, 12]. In another developing nation in Asia, i.e., Bangladesh [13, 14], having the highest population density in the world, almost similar scenario exists. Around 77% of thc population in this country lives in rural areas, and the rural health-care units lack in adequate infrastructure. The population per physician is around 3,000, and population per nurse is around 6,500. The rural health-care centers are sometimes headed by untrained infirmary technicians. In south-Saharan Africa (SSA), the mortality rate of the health-care personnel is another serious issue of concern [15]. The SSA carries 25% of the global burden of disease. In some countries, the death of nurses constitutes almost 40% of annual output from training. The doctor-to-patient ratio is as high as 1:5,000–1:30,000, whereas in developed countries, this is around 1:200–1:500. In [16], an analysis of health infrastructure for two American countries, Peru and Nicaragua, is provided. The study points out that access to major health establishments as one of the major problem, added with little experience of the health staff.

There are two principal modes of telemedicine, viz. real-time interactive mode and 'store and forward' type. In the first case, a real-time feedback is possible by the use of a video link between the 'called' and 'specialty' center by the use of a high-speed dedicated communication link. The expert can consult with the patient-side physician and visually examine the patient. In the other mode, called 'store and forward' type, the patient data is transferred to the consulting hospital using different teletransmission links for storage and offline assessment by experts. The feedback becomes available within a time span of few hours to 3 days.

In most of the developing nations, a three-tire health-care framework is noticed, although the nomenclature varies among the continents. The first and lowermost layer of health-care units is placed in remote rural districts, named primary health-care center (PHC) in India, health posts (HP) in Africa, with non-specialist physicians (sometimes trained/untrained paramedics) and elementary level infrastructure. Most of the PHCs do not have telephone connections and admission facility for long-term checkup. In Asian countries like India, around 100 PHCs are administered by district level hospitals, normally one in each districts, serving around 1–3 million population. The hospitals are having telephone lines, some specialist doctors, better health-care facility, and admission for patient monitoring. The city-based hospitals, residing at highest level, are equipped with specialist doctors, advanced diagnostic and patient monitoring facilities. In case of critical diseases, the patients are referred to city hospitals by rural clinics. However, due to poor connectivity and/or transport facility between rural distracts and urban areas, patients are unable to visit city-based hospitals. The poor health-care infrastructure of remote rural clinics and non-availability of physicians deprive the poor population to get the requisite health-care service in time. As results, mortality rates in districts are many times larger than cities in developing nations.

To address this problem, e-health services through telemedicine technology have been set up in many developing nations to use the ICT for providing the health-care facilities. The basic objective is to connect a rural PHC to a city-based hospital for curative and preventive care of patients through expert advice. Successful implementation of the telemedicine technology requires fulfillment of some basic facilities, given as

1. A dedicated, reliable, cost-effective, and nationwide communication link which will connect the rural clinics with one of the city-based hospitals.
2. Appropriate communication gadgets and compatible health-care/diagnostic equipments for the transmission of patients' pathological data and images through the communication link.
3. Presence of a paramedic or physician at rural health clinic who is conversant with the operation of telemedicine equipments. For city-based hospitals, this is not a big problem since most of the specialist doctors are computer literate.

Among the mentioned issues, the use and implementation of the communication network are the most important criteria, since it is also related to nationwide communication policies of some governments. In Indian scenario, the beginning of telehealth services occurred in mid-1980s. Apollo Telemedicine Enterprises Ltd. (ATEL), a non-profit organization in India, initiated their first modern telemedicine facility at a village called Aragonda in Chitoor district of Andhra Pradesh. In addition to general physicians, some specialist doctors were trained and deployed. The project started with an ultrasound, CT scan, ECHO, an incubator, and automated ECG machine to serve 40 beds of the hospital and a population of 5,000. Connectivity to specialty hospital in Chennai was provided with a simple webcam and ISDN telephone lines. Now the facility equipped with VSAT link caters the need of 24 surrounding villages and a population of 50,000, with specialty centers set up in Hyderabad, Chennai, and other Apollo group of hospitals in India. The 128 kbps ISDN connectivity to Hyderabad is backed up by a 2 Mbps VSAT link. Later on, Sriharikota and Aragonda were directly connected to Chennai specialty center through a VSAT of 2 Mbps connection through Indian Space Research Organization (ISRO). But for all practical reasons, villages can be easily connected using ISDN lines. In the eastern India, Calcutta and Guwahati are two consultation centers that are linked to Hyderabad directly, through a dedicated ISDN line each [17, 18]. A detailed description of telemedicine practice, standards, and protocols used in Indian context is described in [19]. The state of telemedicine in some developing nations is described in [20–23].

Telecardiology, a specialized branch of telemedicine, involves transmission of ECG data and other related information to a remote expert for cardiac checkup. In clinical practice, the ECG data are compressed at the acquisition end to enhance the channel efficiency of the communication link. The practice of telecardiology started early in the nineteenth century when W. Einthoven, the inventor of ECG, investigated the transmission of ECG over telephone lines. This was because the hospital authority did not allow him to remove the patients to his laboratory to test his new device. In India, one of the successful implementations of telecardiology systems was established in Gwalior, India, in 1975 at GR Medical College using an indigenous technique. This system enabled wireless transmission of ECG, using frequency modulation, from the moving ICU van or the patient's home to the central station in ICU of the department of medicine. The ECG output was connected to the telephone input using a modulator, which converted ECG into high-frequency sound. At the other end, a demodulator reconverted the sound into ECG with good gain accuracy. The ECG was converted to sound waves with a frequency varying from 500 to 2,500 Hz with 1,500 Hz at baseline [24]. An advanced system using Internet and database management software developed for telecardiology application for offline analysis by experts is reported [25]. Most of the current practices of telecardiology in Indian health services use either PSTN lines or satellite communication to transfer the compressed ECG files to the referral centers, where the specialists visually examine the ECG records and provide the diagnosis (and the therapy in some occasions) directly (real-time teleconsultation) or by messages (store and forward) to the district hospital.

1.8 Conclusion

Telemedicine assumes special significance in developing nations where the doctor-to-patient ratio is very low. In most of the developing nations, telemedicine practices connect a remote health-care unit to a city-based hospital for real-time teleconsultation, supported by teletransmission of patient's pathological information through dedicated communication links. The development of telemedicine sounds promising to deliver health-care services. Many new initiatives are being observed which uses indigenous techniques toward this effort. Adaptation with new technologies, introduction of user-friendly gadgets, and improved health-care infrastructure can provide a great impetus to telemedicine to serve general population.

Acknowledgments Paper 3 is the contribution from Biomedical Signal acquisition and Processing Research Group at Department of Applied Physics, University of Calcutta, India.

References

1. Katz AM. Physiology of the heart. 5th ed. Philadelphia, PA: Lippincott Williams & Wilkins; 2011.
2. Iaizio PA, editor. Handbook of cardiac anatomy, physiology and devices. 2nd ed. USA: Springer; 2009.
3. Mitra S, Mitra M, Chaudhuri BB. Pattern defined heuristic rules and directional histogram based online ECG parameter extraction. Measurement. 2009;42(1):150–6.

4. Houghton AR, Gray D. Making sense of the ECG: a hands on guide. 3rd ed. UK: Pub Hodder Arnold; 2008.
5. Plonsey R, Fleming DG. Bioelectric phenomena. New York, USA: Mc Graw Hill; 1969.
6. Guler NF, Ubeyli ED. Theory and applications of biotelemetry. J Med Syst. 2002;26(2):159–78.
7. Mackay RS. Bio-medical telemetry: sensing and transmitting biological information from animals and man. Pscataway, NJ: IEEE Press; 1992.
8. Fong B, Fong ACM, Li CK. Telemedicine technologies. West Sussex, UK: Wiley; 2011.
9. http://www.americantelemed.org/.
10. Pal A, Mbarika VWA, Payton FC, Datta P, McCoy S. Telemedicine diffusion in a developing country: the case of India (March 2004). IEEE Tran Inf Tech Biomed. 2005;9(1):59–65.
11. Meethal SP, Jyotish J. A low cost connectivity solution for rural mobile telemedicine. In: IEEE global humanitarian technology conference 2011, 2011, Oct 30–Nov 01, pp. 506–511.
12. Xue Y, Liang H. Analysis of telemedicine diffusion; the case of China. IEEE Tran Inf Tech Biomed. 2007;1(2):231–3.
13. Siddiqua P, Awal MA. A portable telemedicine system in the context of rural Bangladesh. In: IEEE international conference on informatics, electronics and vision, 2012, 18–19 May, Bangladesh, pp. 608–611.
14. Nessa A, Ameen MA, Ullah S, Kwak KS. Applicability of telemedicine in Bangladesh: Current status and future prospects. In: 3rd international conference on convergence and hybrid information technology, 2008, pp. 948–953.
15. Meso P, Mbarika VWA, Sood SP. An overview of potential factors for effective telemedicine transfer to Sub-Saharan Africa. IEEE Tran Inf Tech Biomed. 2009;13(5):734–9.
16. Martinez A, Villarroel V, Seoane J, Pozo F. Analysis of information and communication needs in rural primary healthcare in developing countries. IEEE Tran Inf Tech Biomed. 2005;9(1):66–72.
17. Kumar V, Giri VK, Saxena SC. Telemedicine in context of Indian health scenario. J Inst Eng (I) CP. 2006;87:38–45.
18. Bowonder B, Bansal M, Giridhar AS. A Telemedicine platform: a case study of Apollo hospitals telemedicine project. Int J Serv Technol Manage. 2005;6(3/4/5):449–66.
19. Majumdar AK. Advances in telemedicine and its usage in India. In: International conference on advanced computing and communications (ADCOM), 2007, 18–21 Dec, India, pp. 101–109.
20. Zambrano A, Huerta M, Diaz M, Vivas T (2008) Telemedicine network physical connection design for remote areas, case Baruta- El Hatillo. In: Proceedings of 30th annual international IEEE EMBS conference Vancouver, 2008, British Columbia, Canada, 20–24 Aug, pp. 759–762.
21. Kidiamboko S, Mancini A, Longhi S, Spalazzi L. A scalable telemedicine architecture for underdeveloped countries. A case study: Democratic Republic of Congo. In: Proceedings of 16th mediterranean conference on control and automation congress center, 2008, France, 25–27 June, pp. 866–871.
22. Penjor K, Tshering G, Bhutan health telematics project: overcoming the barriers. In: Proceedings of 6th international workshop on enterprise networking and computing in healthcare industry, HEALTHCOM, 2004, 29 June, pp. 48–53.
23. Irawan YS, Soegijoko S. Development of appropriate telemedicine to improve the management information system for community health care in Indonesia. In: 19th annual IEEE EMBS conference, vol. 3, Chicago, USA, 1997, Oct 30–Nov 2, pp. 991–994.
24. Shanker A, Makhija S, Mantri PK. Teletransmission of ECG waveform: an ingenious low priced technique. Indian Heart J. 1982;34(6):10.
25. Saxena SC, Kumar V, Giri VK. Telecardiology for effective healthcare services. J Med Eng Technol. 2004;27(4):149–59.

Chapter 2
ECG Signal Analysis

2.1 Introduction

This chapter describes the basic steps for analysis of ECG signal using computer-based algorithms. Computerized analysis of ECG started in the early 1960s and considered as one of the first applications of digital computers in medicine. Paper-based long-duration records, while being visually inspected by cardiologists, are susceptible to human errors and suffer from inter-observer variability. Over the decades, numerous ECG analysis algorithms have been developed and tested. There are two prime applications of ECG signal analysis, viz., heart rhythm analysis for continuous ECG monitoring and, ECG feature extraction and classification. Historically, the initial applications used robust computers which were fed with digitized ECG records for automated processing. After the advent of single-chip microprocessors and embedded systems, portable standalone instruments are in use at advanced facilities and ICU setups.

Detailed discussion on different methodologies of ECG analysis is beyond the scope of this book. This chapter describes a brief introduction to ECG signal analysis, followed by a few proposed techniques in time domain.

2.2 Computerized Analysis of ECG

An ECG signal is characterized by sequential repolarization and depolarization of the atria and ventricles, represented by P, QRS, and T waves (with occasional U waves) which are connected by some equipotential segments (PR, ST, and TP). The onset and offset points, along with wave peaks, form a complete basis of delineation of complete wave morphology. Figure 2.1 represents a typical wave sequences P, QRS, and T waves with their respective onset and offset points. Accurate detection of these fiducial points is the first objective of ECG feature extraction. However, the final objective is to compute the ECG clinical signatures, already described in the Sect. 1.4. Among all, the QT interval and the PR

R. Gupta et al., *ECG Acquisition and Automated Remote Processing*,
DOI: 10.1007/978-81-322-1557-8_2,

interval are considered as the most important in the ECG wave. The QT interval is defined as the time from the start of the QRS complex (Q_{on}) to the end of the T wave (i.e., T_{off}) and corresponds to the total duration of electrical activity (both depolarization and repolarization) in the ventricles. Similarly, the PR interval is defined as the time from the start of the P wave (i.e., P_{on}) to the start of the QRS complex (i.e., Q_{on}) and corresponds to the time from the onset of atrial depolarization to the onset of ventricular depolarization. QT interval can provide significant information for diseases related to ventricular activity. Similarly, PR interval can provide information related to AV node conduction problems. Sometimes, the wave shapes and their inclination- or curvature-related parameters also indicate certain diseases, e.g., ST-segment elevation or depression may signify acute myocardial infarction.

Detection of baseline is of paramount importance in case of ECG feature extraction, since all the amplitude features (wave peak heights) are measured with respect to baseline voltage.

The scope of computerized ECG analysis covers R-peak detection for rhythm analysis and feature extraction for disease identification. Accurate detection of ECG fiducial points, P, QRS, and T, and their respective onset and offset points for computation of wave durations along with the heights of wave peaks are the prime objectives of any ECG analysis software. For clinical diagnosis, the cardiologists ask for at least 3–4 cardiac cycles of 12 lead ECG record for visual analysis. For rhythm analysis, however, long-duration (sometimes 24–36 h) ECG records are necessary. In principle, a cardiac cycle can be divided into a low-frequency (P and T waves, and equipotential segments) and high-frequency (QRS complex) regions. In principle, the detection of QRS complex is easier using statistical templates, consisting of slope and amplitude measures. These methods are broadly classified as event detection techniques [1]. In case of ECG signals, however, the presence of different artifacts poses a challenge to the accurate estimation of the position of the fiducial points. Moreover, the shape and magnitude of the ECG vary widely across populations of different continents and determined by food habits, demographic and hereditary factors. Hence, the different algorithms proposed over the years for ECG signal analysis have achieved better accuracy over one another, but none has

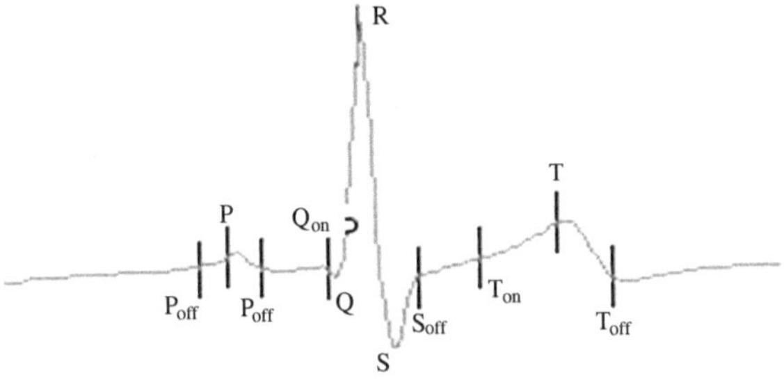

Fig. 2.1 A typical ECG with fiducial points

individually promised 100% perfection level. In general, the steps for ECG signal analysis can be represented by the block diagram shown in Fig. 2.2.

The first step A is normally referred to as 'preprocessing of ECG.' In spite of best practices and precaution during acquisition, ECG signal is corrupted by different types of noises, a brief description of which is provided in Sect. 3.3.1. Among all, power line interference (PLI) [2], baseline wander (BW), and muscle tremor (EMG noise) are dominant in affecting the ECG wave shapes. A detailed discussion on motion artifacts, power line interference, electrosurgical interference, and their minimizing techniques are discussed in [3].

QRS being the sharpest and steep region in the ECG cycle is relatively easy to detect, and hence, Step B is most important. Many cardiac signal analysis algorithms start with this step in order to capture other wave peaks with respect to already-detected R peaks. Once the fiducial points are detected, the wave signatures can be computed by simple mathematical steps. Since the wave signatures of a normal person also vary slightly among the beats in continuous recording, Step D and E are used to identify the variance of clinical signatures among the different beats by statistical calculation.

Fig. 2.2 Generalized steps for ECG signal analysis

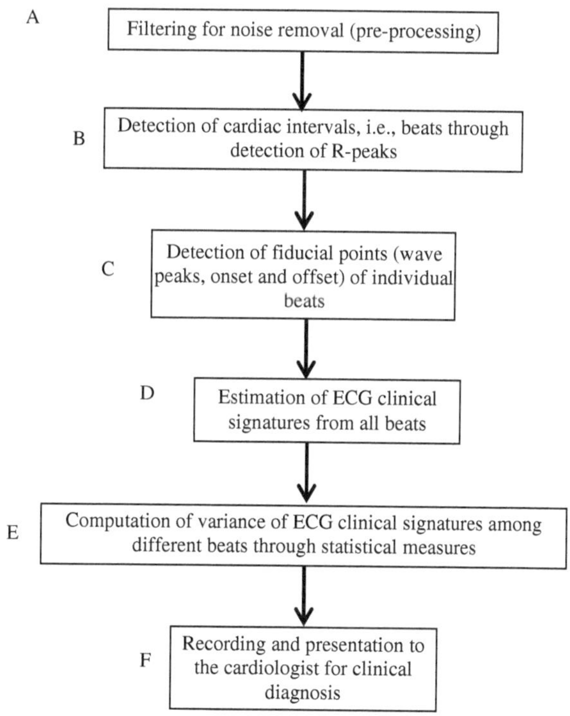

In the following sections, a brief review of ECG analysis algorithms are provided, divided into three parts, viz., preprocessing methodologies, R-peak detection techniques and feature extraction techniques.

2.3 Review on Computerized ECG Processing Techniques

2.3.1 Denoising Techniques

ECG denoising is aimed to eliminate (or, at least minimize) the unwanted signals from an ECG record, without hampering the clinical information contained within the signal itself. A detailed review of the denoising methods is available in [4]. The available literature on ECG denoising mostly discusses PLI and BW removal. In many reported works, the researchers have validated the algorithm by introducing a simulated noise with a 'clean' ECG signal to generate a composite noisy signal and then denoising it using their proposed algorithm.

In general, the ECG denoising techniques can be classified into one of the following categories:

(a) Digital filtering techniques—adaptive and non-adaptive;
(b) Source separation methods—principal component analysis (PCA) and independent component analysis (ICA);
(c) Neural networks;
(d) Wavelet-based methods;
(e) Other non-adaptive methods like empirical mode decomposition (EMD), etc.

The early approaches for noise filtering, prior to 1980s, were based on digital filters [5]. For computerized processing of ECG, the recommendation for filtering bandwidths and other specifications is guided by AHA circulation [6]. Design of a digital filter with integer coefficients for microprocessor implementation is reported [7]. The paper analyzes the performance and errors due to quantization, rounding-off operation of the filter coefficients, their representation, and overflow while implemented in NSC800 and 680E52 microprocessors. Using sampling rate of 360 Hz, a comparative analysis of non-adaptive and adaptive notch filters for PLI reduction is carried out in [8] in terms of computational efficiency (number of multiplications), distortion of the signal, and residual signal entropy. The adaptive filter implemented by Tompkins et al. [9] with an internally generated reference was found to be efficient than the non-adaptive counterpart. A common problem with the notch filter is the transient response which affects its performance for real-time operations. Reference [10] deals a technique for suppression of transient responses at the expenses of some computational load in the initial stages. A new adaptive technique for PLI reduction is described in [11] where the line interference signal on the patient body is separately recorded using a hardware arrangement. A common problem with linear phase filtering is large number of multiplications which result in long computation time. The method described in [12] enhances the computational efficiency by reducing the number of impulse response coefficients and using the symmetry of the impulse response. The prescribed method reduced the number of coefficients by a factor of 5 compared to conventional NRFIR filter and halved the number of multiplications. Application of adaptive filtering for noise cancelation is described in [13]. Different types of adaptive filter structures, viz., basic adaptive filter, least mean square (LMS) algorithm, and adaptive recurrent filter (ARF), are applied for reduction in power line interference, EMG, motion artifact, and BW in ambulatory ECG monitoring. A cascaded adaptive filter for removal of BW is described [14], and its performance is compared with cubic spline approach [15] while applied to MIT-BIH arrhythmia database. The proposed method used an adaptive zero frequency notch filter followed by adaptive impulse correlated filter (AICF). Conventional BW removal methods using band-pass filter (0.05–100 Hz) suffer from the disadvantages that they distort the ECG at two distinct frequencies, viz., 0 Hz (ideal baseline voltage) and 0.8 Hz [16]. A new adaptive filter, which is a combination of time-sequenced adaptive filter (TSAF) and AICF, is proposed in [17]. Morphological operators have been widely used in the signal and image processing domains because of their robust and adaptive performance in extracting the shape information in addition to their simple and quick set computation. Morphological filters are based on some mathematical structures which capture the structural property of the signal by applying a set of structural element on the dataset. A modified Morphological operator-based ECG filtering technique is described in [18]. Adaptive noise cancelation provides a means for a no priory knowledge of the signal or the noise characteristics. In this technique [19], two input signals are fed to the noise canceler block. The first input is called the 'primary,' containing the corrupted signal, i.e., signal plus noise. The second one is called 'reference,' contains the noise correlated with some way with the primary noise. This noise is filtered to make a close replica with the primary noise. The outputs are subtracted to produce the noise-free signal. An adaptive Kalman filtering technique is proposed in [20] for baseline removal from the ECG signal. The ECG is simulated as a piecewise linear triangular function, smoothed by third-order Savitzky-Golay FIR filter. The baseline is generated by a second-order polynomial.

PCA is a statistical tool that decorrelates the different signal components from ECG data [21], while ICA considers the noise signals as independent entity in the ECG signal. [22] deals with PCA followed by different versions of ICA application for ECG segmentation and QRS detection, noise reduction in CSE database. In [23], a modification of classical PCA, named 'projection pursuit approach,' is used for ECG enhancement with the objective of analysis of ECG beat variability.

An artificial neural network (ANN) is an interconnected chain of computational units (nodes) that simulates a human brain for its ability of learning from the data. A neural net is trained with known similar datasets which it used to gather knowledge about the data. With an unknown dataset, the network responds better from its acquired knowledge. An application of NN-based adaptive filter in wavelet domain for noise removal is reported in [24]. A wavelet-based optimal filter is designed where the filter weights are optimized by an unbiased linear ANN. Here, the network weights related to each wavelet sub-band are computed by steepest deepest algorithm. A new technique with reduced number of hidden layers and less computational time by using An MADALINE (Multiple ADAptive LINear Element) structure is reported to eliminate white, artifact sand muscular noise in [25].

Wavelet-based multiresolution analysis is one of the popular methods for ECG denoising in recent times, due to its excellent time frequency resolution properties. Using discrete wavelet transform (DWT), the signal can be resolved in different frequency bands from which a combination of different coefficients can be utilized for identification noise components and eliminating them, in principle, to get a clean signal. In [26, 27] the authors propose a dyadic DWT decomposition using Daubechie's wavelet and discard appropriate coefficients in the decomposition layer and reconstruct the signal to get a fairly accurate results. The methods provide a quick and easy removal method for BW and muscle noise. Wavelet-based denoising can effectively reject the noisy components. In wavelet-based thresholding methods, the coefficients after wavelet decomposition are adjusted by use of a threshold that can either be set as 'hard' or 'soft.' In 'hard' thresholding, the coefficient values below the threshold are set to zero, thus, eliminating the noise associated with those components of the signal. In 'soft' thresholding, the values below the threshold are reduced by the same magnitude from their original values. The processed coefficients are then reconstructed back to the time domain to get a noise-free signal. In [28], a non-linear denoising approach was proposed by applying soft and hard thresholding methods, in which thresholds were chosen using four different methods, viz., 'Stein's unbiased risk estimate' (SURE) [29], heuristic SURE (HEUR-SURE), fixed threshold (FIX-THRES), and MINIMAX [30]. An application of wavelet thresholding method for EMG noise removal is described in [31], and the results are compared with Vapnik–Chervonenkis (VC) learning theory, which is related to statistical learning theory and to empirical processes. Some more applications of wavelet-based denoising are available [32–34].

EMD proposed by Huang et al. is one of the fully data-driven techniques used for non-linear and non-stationery signals and does not require *a priory* knowledge of the signal. The EMD process defines a signal into a sum of intrinsic mode functions (IMF), with equal number of extrema and zero crossing with its envelope, symmetric with respect to zero. The signal is reconstructed by eliminating the IMFs which correspond to frequency components, similar to DWT approach [35]. In [36], the authors also deal with the problem that arises due to truncation of R peaks resulting out of direct elimination of IMFs during reconstruction by introducing a 'peak correction method.'

The common performance parameters used for noise removal from the ECG are given as

$$\begin{aligned} \text{Mean Square Error (MSE)} &= \frac{1}{N}\sum_{i=1}^{N}\left[x(i)-\tilde{x}(i)\right]^2 \\ \text{Signal to Noise Ratio (SNR)} &= 10 \times \log\frac{\sum x^2(i)}{\sum n^2(i)} \\ \text{Percentage Root Mean Square Difference (PRD)} &= \sqrt{\frac{\sum\left[x(i)-\tilde{x}(i)\right]^2}{\sum x^2(i)}} \end{aligned} \tag{2.1}$$

where N is the total number of samples, x is the clean sample, n is the known noise, and $\tilde{x}$ is the denoised sample. Some authors have also estimated a few indirect measures, viz., percentage noise retention ratio (PNR) [36], noise reduction factors (NRF) [37], and SNR improvement, defined as

$$\begin{aligned} \text{Percentage Noise Retention (PNR)} &= \frac{P_{\text{ds}} - P_{\text{cs}}}{P_{\text{cs}}} \times 100 \\ \text{Noise Reduction Factor (NRF)} &= \sqrt{\frac{\sum\left[\hat{x}(i) - x(i)\right]^2}{\sum\left[\tilde{x}(i) - x(i)\right]^2}} \\ \text{SNR Improvement (SNR imp) [dB]} = \text{SNR}_i - \text{SNR}_O &= 10 \times \log\frac{\sum_i \frac{x^2(i)}{n^2(i)}}{\sum_i \frac{x^2(i)}{\left[\tilde{x}(i) - x(i)\right]^2}} \end{aligned} \tag{2.2}$$

where $P = 10 \times \log\sum|x(i)|^2$; P_{cs} denotes the power of the clean signal, and P_{DS} the same of the denoised signal, $\hat{x}$ is the composite (noisy) signal with the clean ECG, $\tilde{x}(i) - x(i)$ is the residual noise. SNR_i and SNR_o denote the SNR at input and output, respectively.

2.3.2 R-peak Detection Methods

The rhythm statements of ECG can be obtained from the R-peak locations. Due to its characteristic shape, QRS complex is the most prominent part of an ECG wave. For this reason, R-peak detection is taken up as the starting point of many ECG analysis algorithms. Typically, the QRS wave frequency is in the range 10–25 Hz. Ideally, a band-pass filter with upper and lower cutoff frequencies at these levels applied to ECG signal would reveal the QRS. However, the wide variation of QRS morphologies and the presence of noise makes it difficult to identify the QRS is abnormal heart signals. Till date, numerous QRS detection algorithms have been reported and successfully tested. However, no reported work has achieved absolute accuracy for all diseases. Normally, QRS detection is indicated by R-peak locations (QS peak for positive R-wave absent). The measures of QRS detection by software are described by the following parameters [38]:

$$\text{Sensitivity } (S_e) = \frac{\text{TP}}{\text{TP} + \text{FN}}$$
$$\text{Positive Predictivity } (P+) = \frac{\text{TP}}{\text{TP} + \text{FP}} \tag{2.5}$$

where the first letter describes the correctness of the detection algorithm (i.e., right or wrong) in terms of TRUE or FALSE. The second letter indicates the output of the algorithm (i.e., found or not found) in terms of POSITIVE or NEGATIVE. For example, TP (true positive) stands for correctly detected peaks, FN (false negative) for missed peaks and FP (false positive) for misdetections. Sometimes, a third parameter named, specificity (S_p), is used, defined as

$$\text{Specificity } (S_p) = \frac{\text{TN}}{\text{TN} + \text{FP}} \tag{2.6}$$

where TN (true negative) stands for a correctly detected non-QRS region. The four conditions can be described by the chart shown in Table 2.1.

The QRS detection algorithms can be classified into the following classes:

(a) Principles based on digital filters and derivatives;
(b) Template matching techniques;
(c) Wavelet and other non-linear transform-based approaches;
(d) Neural network and GA techniques.

A typical software-based QRS detector can be represented by Fig. 2.3. The first stage, called 'preprocessing stage,' eliminates the noises and enhances the QRS features. The following stage applies the peak detection logic based on some rules and characterizes it.

A comprehensive review and comparison of QRS detection algorithms are provided in [39]. The early approaches for QRS detection (up to 1985) used discrete-derivative-based methods [40] based on digital filters, implemented

Table 2.1 Interpretation of sensitivity parameters

	True	False
Positive	Wave peak (R) is correctly detected at its position	Wave peak is detected at other positions (misdetected)
Negative	Wave peak is not found in non-QRS region	Wave peak is missed at correct position

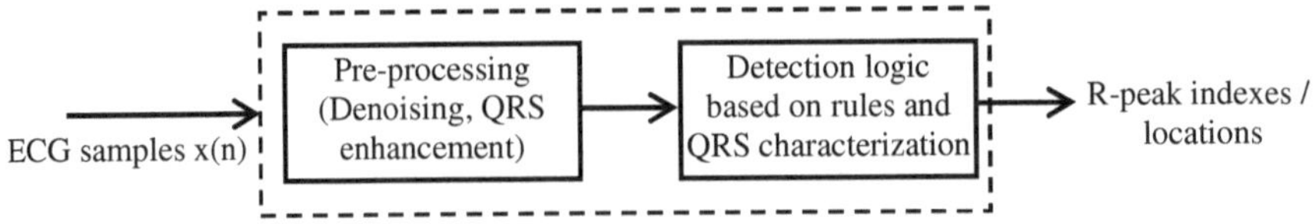

Fig. 2.3 Generalized software-based QRS detection representation

through difference equations in microcomputer-based systems for Holter tape analysis [41, 42]. An arrhythmia detection algorithm based on filtering, differentiation, energy collector, and a classifier is described [43]. This algorithm generated a delay of 1 s while implemented in real time with 250-Hz sampling. Pan Tompkins algorithm [44] is considered as one of the early pioneering works of microprocessor-based real-time QRS detection and provided benchmark for performance analysis for other researchers during the following decades. The algorithm is based on digital analysis of slope, amplitude, and width and QRS energy. The algorithm was implemented on Zilog 80 microprocessor, with a very good accuracy (total detection failure of 0.67%) with 487 records. The improved version of this algorithm [45] showed an improved performance (99.68% sensitivity and 99.63% predictivity) based on an event detector from the preprocessing stage of QRS detection. In [46], a comparison between the first-derivative-based methods, especially Pan Tompkins, Hamilton-Tompkins with Hilbert transform (HT) methods, is drawn.

In [47], an adaptive algorithm based on maximum a posteriori (MAP) estimation is described. A mathematical model of pulse-shaped waveform for QRS detection is developed, and its estimation procedure is estimated. To adapt with varying QRS morphology, the detector (estimator) adjusts the parameters with incoming beats. In [48], the same model as in [47] is dealt with; however, a simplification in the model is introduced.

QRS detection using mathematical morphology is described in [49]. In this approach, a morphological operator followed by peak value extractor (PVE), which suppresses the non-QRS regions and converts the QRS peaks into sharp complexes. Finally, an adaptive threshold-based rule base determines the QRS locations. A mathematical operator based on morphology of the QRS complex is described in [50]. A new concept of dominant wavelet rescaled coefficients (DWRC) is used, where the relation between QRS complex and their corresponding wavelet coefficients is derived analytically. In the model, a typical ECG beat is approximated as summation of two sinus functions as P and T waves and three triangles as QRS complex. A morphology alignment method for using a piecewise uniform re-sampling ECG waveform is prescribed in [51]. A heartbeat is first delineated into stable and flexible segments. These segments are then resampled at two different rates such that re-sampling frequency becomes uniform for the same segments in all beats. The morphological features extracted from each heartbeat are evaluated for alignment of an ideal morphology.

A number of non-linear transformations for QRS detection are available in literature. Among them, [52] described a multiplication of backward difference (MOBD) operator to multiply the successive differences to feed in a decision rule based on adaptive threshold to detect the QRS regions. The HT [53] for QRS detection is proposed in [54]. The first difference of the signal is computed and its HT is used to detect the point of inflexions in waveform, which appears as peak in HT dataset. Then, an adaptive threshold based on statistical parameters of the Hilbert sequence is used for detecting R peaks.

Suitability of wavelet transforms for non-stationery biomedical signal analysis, especially ECG, was established by a number of publications in the 1990s. Due to the multiresolution property of the wavelet transform, it has been used in the efficient detection of QRS complexes. Many of the reported works are based on Mallat's and Hwang's approach for singularity detection using local maxima of the wavelet coefficient signal [55–57]. In [55], a spline wavelet developed for varying QRS morphology is proposed. The dyadic wavelet transform (D_yWT) was computed using a wavelet which is the first derivative of a smoothing function. It exhibited local maxima at the QRS occurrences. A continuous wavelet transform is proposed in [56] to detect QRS. The algorithm used first-order derivative to suppresses the noise and baseline drift and high-scale continuous wavelet transform to pick the zero crossing R point produced by differentiator to ease the task of QRS detection. In the proposed method, at first, a 3-point moving-window integrator is used for low-pass filtering, followed by a first-order derivative to eliminate baseline drift and muscle noise. Finally, CWT is used for QRS detection. In [57], a CWT implementation is shown using DSP processor for real-time detection of ECG characteristic points.

Artificial neural networks and other intelligent computational techniques are in use for ECG analysis, especially arrhythmia monitoring [58]. In [59] an adaptive matched filter is proposed whose coefficients are updated by an ANN. A multilayer perceptron (MLP) neural network structure is used for an adaptive whitening filter. The QRS template used for matched filtering is updated by an ANN recognition algorithm, which provides better adaptation to signal changes. A new method, employing multichannel adaptive resonance theory (MART) neural network is described in [60] for efficient QRS detection. An FIR filter based on Keiser window is adopted for removal of PLI and BLW from the ECG. The R peaks are initially detected by 32-point averaging and peak detection method. The RS segment is approximated by a side of a triangle of variable width for training the network. The Mart network uses two channels of data for detection of Q and S points. In [61], a genetic design for QRS detection is described. At the first stage, a linear polynomial filter is used for QRS enhancement. In order to operate on small number of input samples, a genetic algorithm-based optimization of filter coefficients is performed, which only detect the maxima of the filtered output and ignores QRS like spikes.

2.3.3 Feature Extraction from ECG Signal

Computerized ECG feature extractions are aimed to delineate the complete waveforms from the ECG dataset. A detailed survey of different ECG feature extraction techniques are discussed in [62, 63]. In general, the feature extraction techniques are classified into the following:

(a) Time-domain methods based on morphology and adaptive filtering;

(b) Time-frequency analysis using wavelet and other non-linear transforms;
(c) PCA, neural networks, and other methods.

Computerized interpretation of electrocardiogram is started in the early 1960 with the introduction of digital computers in the USA by Caceres et al. In [64], a tele-transmission and computerized processing is described. The data acquisition from the patient was done in a portable ECG machine, coupled with a patient coder and FM tape recorder by a technician. The incoming ECG was recorded and processed by an IBM 360/50 computer. The system showed fairly accurate result acceptable to cardiologists. Later on, in the 1970s, microprocessor standalone units were in use for automated interpretation. In [65], use of a microcomputer-based 3-channel ECG analysis system for P wave, arrhythmia, and axis analysis is described. In [66], a time-domain morphology and gradient-based algorithm is presented. The algorithm is based on a combination of extrema detection and slope information, with the use of adaptive thresholding to achieve the extraction of 11 number of time instances. These 11 time signatures are onset and offset points of waves and wave peaks. After the initial QRS detection, the onset and offset of QRS are detected, by considering them as points of maximum or minimum electrical activity around them. From the S-offset T, T-onset, and T-off set are detected by a zonal search of appropriate width imposed with slope-based criteria. To detect the wave peaks in 'double humped' cases, adaptive threshold values are used to enhance the detection accuracy. A statistical method based on comparison of relative magnitudes of ECG samples and their slope in time domain is described in [67]. In [68], an investigation on detecting the boundaries of P and T wave is carried out using the LMS algorithm. The authors propose an adjustment of the adaptation constant imposed with an extreme condition to determine the end of T wave. A morphology-based ECG heartbeat classifier is reported in [69, 70]. From a training data using MIT-BIH arrhythmia dataset, a set of 12 features are selected based on ECG morphology, heartbeat intervals, and RR intervals. After the pre-processing for noise elimination, heartbeats are segmented followed by fiducial point detection. Linear discriminants (LDs) were used to operate on heartbeat interval features and segmented ECG morphology features. A similar study [71] used Kohonen self-organizing maps (SOM) and linear vector quantization algorithms to operate on ANSI/AAMI EC57 standard data.

Use of wavelet transform for ECG characterization is described [72–74]. In [75], the QRS detection is performed by modulus maxima of wavelet transform. The modulus maxima of a normal biphasic QRS are also biphasic. Hence, an adjustable threshold is used to select the QRS in the scale of 21–24 in wavelet transform. The QRS-onset and QRS-offset are selected at first modulus maxima pair. The onset and offset of P and T waves are searched in the scale of 2^3. The P wave searched in a 200-ms window ahead of Q-onset, and for T wave, the same procedure is adopted after S-offset. The algorithm is implemented on a TMS 320C25 DSP which accesses 12-lead ECG at a 16-bit resolution and sampling of

500 Hz. Use of HT in ECG analysis is described in [76, 77]. A unique property of the transform that the transformed output undergoes a polarity change (i.e., crosses over x axis) whenever the original wave has a slope reversal point. In a typical ECG waveform, the slope reversal ideally occurs at the fiducial points. However, the original waveform is required to be preprocessed to remove the noise for proper detection. PCA has been used for minimization of feature space data extracted through DWT decomposition using db4 as mother wavelet [78]. A short-time Fourier transform (STFT) along with Gabor filter is utilized for R-peak detection and feature extraction within the QRS zone [79]. In [80], a MLP ANN has been used for classifying the features of ECG detected through discrete Fourier transform (DFT), PCA, and DWT.

2.4 Method of ECG Signal Analysis

In this section, a few simple methods of ECG signal analysis is described in the sequence: ECG preprocessing, QRS detection, and ECG feature extraction. The data analysis algorithm is applied on a single-lead ECG data from Physionet database (ptb data and mit-db data). At first, all the R peaks are determined from the data. We propose three different methods for R-peak detection, viz., (a) differential ECG with slope-based criteria, (b) square derivative with amplitude threshold-based search, and (c) amplitude span with slope-based criteria. Next, the baseline positions are detected in the TP segment of each beat, and baseline modulated is corrected by an empirical formula. Finally, each wave peaks and their respective onset and offset points are detected with respect to R-peak locations. Finally, the time-plane features are computed. The steps of ECG data analysis are represented by Fig. 2.4.

The preprocessing of ECG can be done by any suitable method as described in the Sect. 2.3.1. In the proposed feature extraction methods, ECG data from Physionet has been used. For R-peak detection, MIT-BIH arrhythmia data (mitdb)

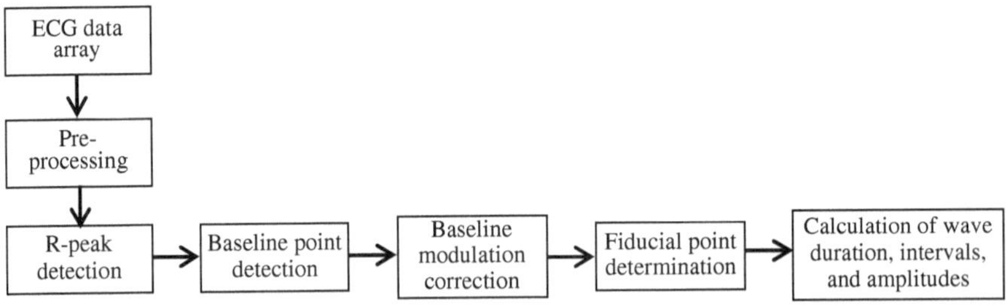

Fig. 2.4 ECG data analysis steps

and PTB-Diagnostic ECG data (ptbdb) have been used. For feature extraction, only the ptbdb data have been used.

2.4.1 QRS Detection

2.4.1.1 Processing of Differential ECG Data

Normally, the region of QRS is with highest slope (or, inter-sample difference) in a typical ECG beat. A method of QRS detection is developed by processing of differential ECG or D-ECG, which is generated by computing the successive sample differences of the ECG samples. From an ECG data array x, the corresponding D-ECG array y is generated as

$$y(i) = x(i + 1) - x(i) \tag{2.10}$$

Since the maximum width of QRS region is nominally 96 ms, a window of same width is slid along the D-ECG array to find out a probable QRS neighborhood by use of some criteria. The objective is to capture an index near to the sharp peak in order to reveal QRS region. At this index, the following criteria must match the following:

1. Absolute value of sample will be greater than or equal to 50 % of maximum sample magnitude;
2. Average slope, computed over ±3 samples around will be positive;
3. Average slope, computed over ±3 samples around at 30 points downside will be negative;
4. Mean absolute slope will be greater than or equal to 30 % of maximum absolute slope of the D-ECG array.

Matching all these criteria would locate a sample on the rising edge of an R peak, named as 'R-threshold point' as shown in Fig. 2.5. Then, from this 'R-threshold point,' next 50 upside samples are sorted in descending order of their magnitude as well as index. The position of highest amplitude is provisionally taken as the R peak. Its candidature is cross-verified by a slope sign reversal within 50 samples upside along the array from this point. For ECG records with QS

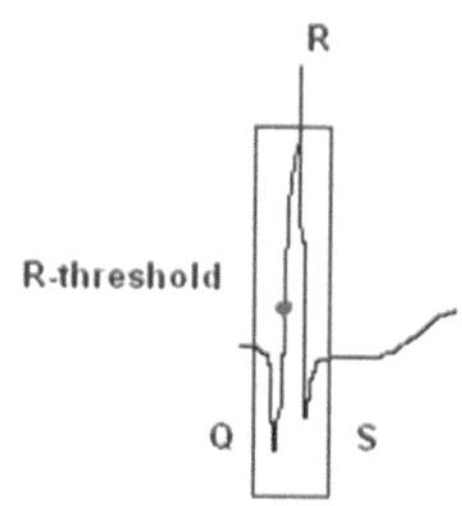

Fig. 2.5 R-threshold point

Table 2.2 S_e and P+ figures for ptb-db using differential ECG

Patient file ID and record No. in Physionet	Lead I		Lead II		Lead III		Lead aVR		Lead V1		Lead V3	
	S_e	P+	S_e	P+	S_e	P+	S_e	P+	S_e	P+	S_e	P+
P245/s0480 (N)	100	100	100	100	100	100	100	100	100	100	100	100
P248/s0481 (N)	100	100	100	100	100	100	100	100	100	100	100	100
P249/s0484 (M)	100	100	100	100	100	100	100	100	100	100	100	100
P092/s0354 (MI-Inf)	100	100	100	100	100	100	100	100	80.1	87.2	100	100
P092/s0358(MI-Inf)	100	100	100	100	100	100	100	100	100	100	100	100
P093/s0378 (MI-Inf)	100	100	100	100	100	100	100	100	100	100	100	100
P002/0015(MI-Ant)	100	100	100	100	100	100	100	100	100	100	80.7	85
P056/0196 (MI-Ant)	100	100	94.8	100	100	85	100	100	100	100	75	75
P262/s0498 (C)	100	100	100	100	100	100	100	100	100	100	100	100
P287/s0548 (Inf-post-lat))	100	100	100	100	100	100	100	100	100	100	100	100

Narration N Normal; *M* Myocarditis; *MI* Myocardial infarction; *Ant* Anterior; *Inf* Inferior; *C* Cardiomyopathy; *Inf-post-lat* Inferio posterio lateral

Table 2.3 S_e and P+ figures for mit-db using differential ECG

Patient ID and lead number from Physionet	S_e	P+
100 (v5)	100	100
101 (v1)	98.53	100
102 (v2)	100	100
103 (v2)	100	100
107 (v2)	100	100
112 (v1)	100	100
113 (v1)	98.11	100
114 (ML-II)	100	100

peaks, the slope reversal would not take place, and so, the sample within the window having lowest magnitude is taken as the QRS peak.

Condition (4) eliminates the possibility of misdetection of P or T peak as R peak. For ECG data with QS peaks, this would locate the QS region. The algorithm steps are given in the end of the chapter Appendix 1. Some test results using PhysioNet data the method is shown in Tables 2.2 and 2.3. Figure 2.6a and b shows R-peak detection, baseline modulation correction using ptb-db and mit-db data respectively.

2.4.1.2 Using Square Derivative with Amplitude Threshold Criteria

The approach is primarily aimed to reveal the sharp slope changes in the QRS region of the ECG data. Since the slope changes can have positive as well as negative values, at first, the sample array is squared to enhance the QRS regions

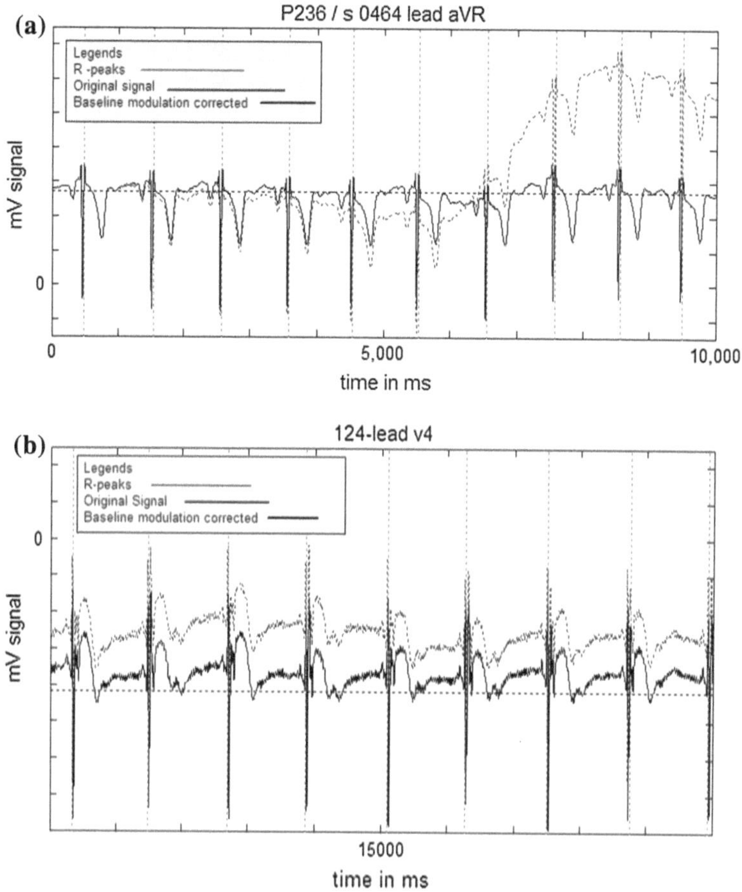

Fig. 2.6 R-peak detection from using differential ECG. **a** using ptb-db data, **b** using mit-db data

and then first and second derivative of the data are computed. In this approach, numerical differentiation using Lagrange's five-point interpolation formula is used. According to [81], five-point derivative prevents high-frequency noise amplification. The formula used is given in Eq. 2.11.

$$f_0' = \frac{1}{12h}(f_{-2} - 8f_{-1} + 8f_1 - f_2) \tag{2.11}$$

where index '0' indicates current sample of reference and others are with respect to the current position index, h refers to the tolerance level.

Figure 2.7 shows the original signal, with squared first- and second-derivative plot. The squared signal after second derivative sharply localizes QRS regions. The exact location of R peak is determined by a window search as follows:

Table 2.4 S_e and P+ figures for Ptb-db using squared derivative approach

Patient file ID and record no. in Physionet	Lead I	Lead III	Lead aVR	Lead V1	Lead V3
P236/s0462 (N)	96.29	100	85.71	100	100
P236/s0463 (N)	100	100	85.71	100	100
P246/s0478 (N)	100	71.05	100	100	100
P247/s0479 (N)	98.91	97.23	100	97.23	95.45
P248/s0481 (N)	100	100	96.55	100	100
P249/s0484 (M)	100	96.3	100	100	100
P265/s0501 (Ant-Lat)	100	100	100	100	100
P092/s0354 (MI-Inf)	100	98.52	99.24	97.56	98.12
P092/s0358 (MI-Inf)	96.11	98.42	99.12	100	100
P093/s375 (MI-Inf)	100	100	100	100	100
P262/s0498 (C)	100	100	100	100	100

Narration N Normal; *M* Myocarditis; *MI* Myocardial infarction; *Ant* Anterior; *Inf* Inferior; *C* Cardiomyopathy

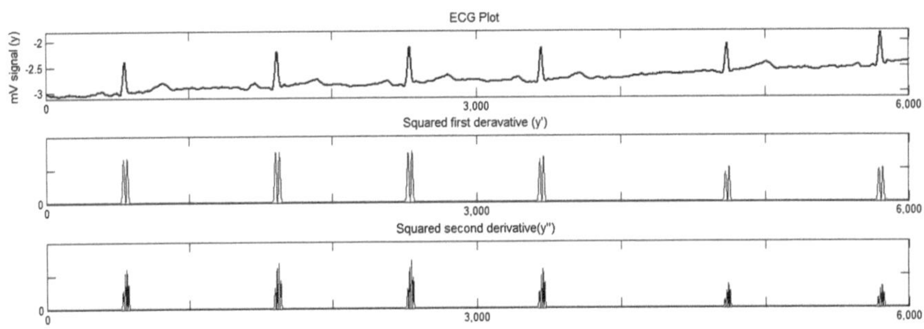

Fig. 2.7 R-peak detection using squared derivative approach

At first, the sample with highest second-derivative squared (say $d2'$ array) is located. Let this value is $d2$ max. Since the normal QRS region is around 96 ms, a search in the original dataset (say, $y2$) around $\pm$ 45-ms window for highest value would yield the R peak. This R peak is the sharpest R peak of the dataset. The other QRS regions are found out by a search in the $d2'$ dataset by locating samples which exceed a preset threshold value (say, 5%) of the $d2$ max magnitude. Starting from each of these index points, the corresponding R peak is determined as the sample with highest magnitude within a $\pm$45-ms window in the original data array. Once all the R peaks are determined, their indexes are taken in an array and average R–R interval is computed. The related algorithm steps are given in the end of the chapter Appendix 2. Figure 2.8a and b shows R-peak detection, baseline modulation correction using ptb-db and mit-db data, respectively. Some test results with ptb-db data are shown is table 2.4.

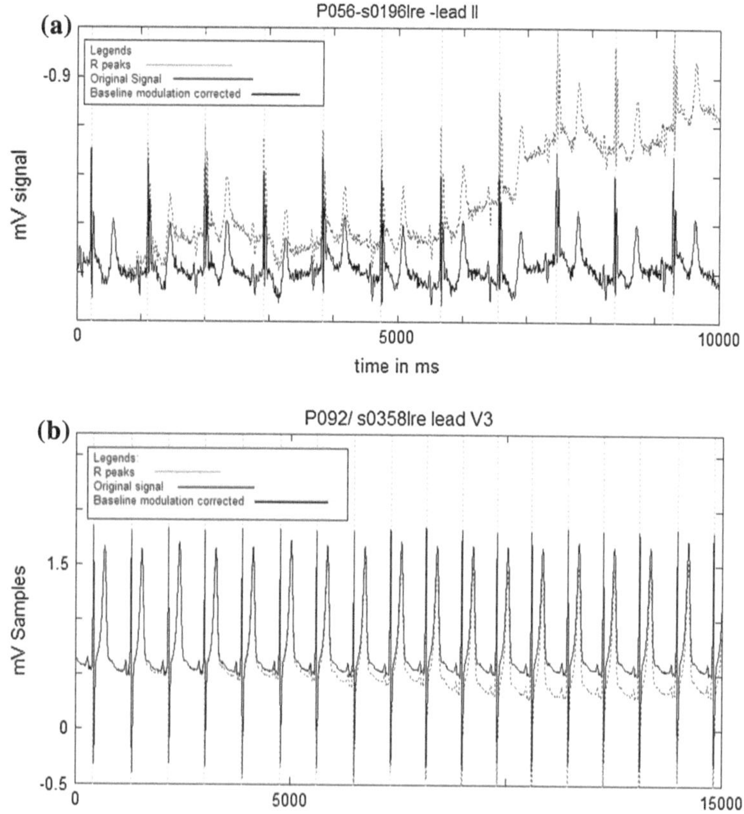

Fig. 2.8 R-peak detection from using squared derivative ECG. **a** using ptb-db data(MI-*anterior*), **b** using ptb-db data(MI-*inferior*)

2.4.1.3 Using Amplitude Span Detection of QRS Region

In this technique, the QRS detection is based on the following features in a typical ECG dataset.

1. The QRS segment width is nominally 96 ms, within which, Q (or S) peak to R peak maximum distance is 60 ms;
2. Slope change in the QRS region is the maximum;
3. For a particular lead, the QRS amplitude span, defined as the vertical distance between R-peak ordinate to the same of Q peak (or S peak), remains almost constant throughout the dataset.

A sliding window of 96-ms width is moved by 20 ms in steps through the entire dataset to form a rule base which is used for detecting the QRS templates. Thus, the total process is divided into two stages, viz., rule-base generation and QRS detection. At first, the following parameters are computed for the entire dataset using the 96-ms window, slid with a step of 20 ms:

1. Maximum QRS amplitude span in 96-ms window;
2. Maximum 8-point average positive slope (inter-sample difference).

This captures the tallest and sharpest QRS in the dataset.

The following rules for QRS neighborhood are fixed as: (1) amplitude span in moving 96-ms window should exceed 80% of maximum amplitude span computed over same window span. Let this value be $span_{th}$. This rule is named as 'amplitude threshold' criteria (ATC). (2) Average (8-point) slope should exceed 80% of maximum average slope (say, mx_slp) computed over dataset in a moving 96 samples. Let this value be slp_{th}. This rule is named as 'slope threshold' criteria (STC).

Now, from the beginning of the ECG dataset, a fresh search is initiated in a sliding 96-ms window with step of 20 ms to meet $span_{th}$ criteria. This may locate a probable QRS neighborhood. This is shown in Fig. 2.9. It is also concluded that to

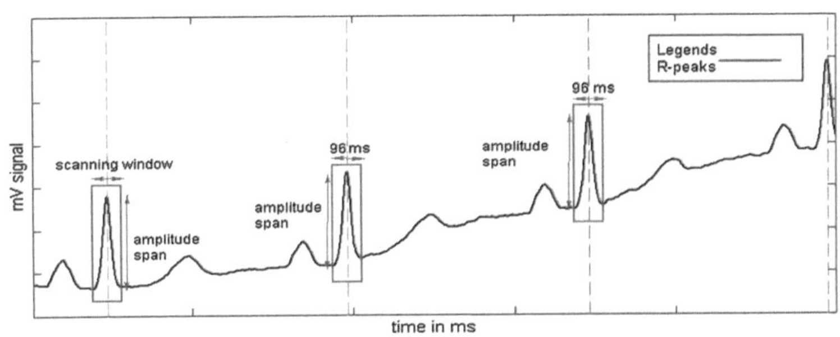

Fig. 2.9 QRS detection by sliding window

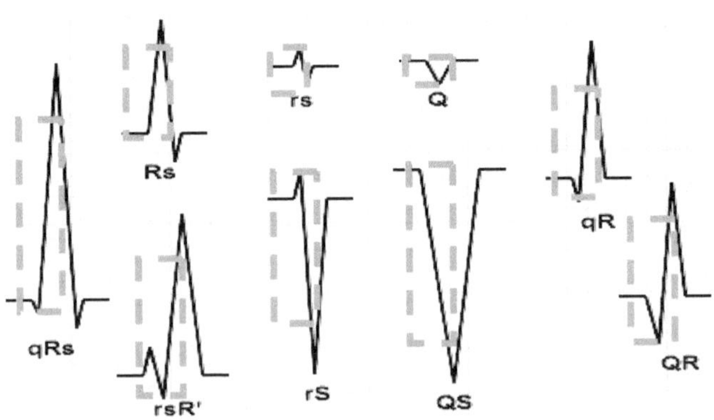

Fig. 2.10 Different QRS types captured by 96-ms window

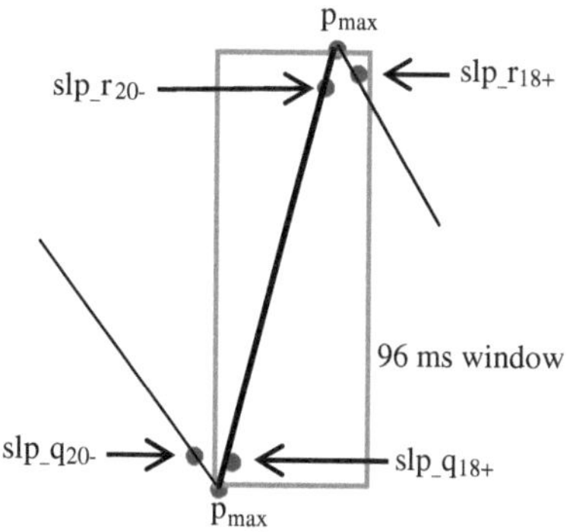

Fig. 2.11 Finding slope inversion across maximum and minimum point in a 96-ms window

match ATC, this window may contain either R or Q or S peak as its local maxima or minima, or even tall T peak for some ECG records.

Figure 2.10 represents some of the possibilities of different QRS shapes which may be captured by moving 96-ms window. Now, from this position, any of the R or Q or S peak within this window is determined by a direction-based slope sign reversal search initiated from the local maxima or minima, as illustrated with Fig. 2.11.

This is determined as follows:

Let $p_{\max}$ and $p_{\min}$ are the indexes of maximum and minimum points in a 96-ms window. Then, 16-point average slope at 20 samples downside (i.e., decreasing index) and 18 samples upside (i.e., index increasing) at $p_{\max}$ and $p_{\min}$ is calculated. Let these values be:

$$\begin{array}{c}\text{for}\, p_{\max}\text{:}\ \text{slp\_}r_{20-},\ \text{slp\_}r_{18+}, \quad \text{and} \quad \text{for}\, p_{\min}:\ \text{slp\_}q_{20-}\ \text{and}\, \text{slp\_}q_{18+}. \\ \text{if}\, \text{slp\_}r_{20-}\ > 0 \quad \text{and} \quad \text{slp\_}r_{18+} < 0\end{array} \tag{2.12}$$

we may conclude that there is a slope sign reversal near to $p_{\max}$

$$\text{and}\, \text{if}\, \text{slp\_}q_{20-} < 0 \quad \text{and} \quad \text{slp\_}q_{18+} > 0 \tag{2.13}$$

we conclude that there is a slope sign reversal near to $p_{\min}$.

Both Eqs. (2.12) and (2.13) may also be satisfied in a moving 96-ms window. But it does not ensure a neighborhood of R peak, since a positive or negative T peak may also satisfy Eqs. (2.12) and (2.13) respectively. To determine the correct position of QRS, rule (2), i.e., STC criteria is used.

For Eqs (2.12) or (2.13) being satisfied, a new window of 96 ms is formed around $p_{\max}$ (or $p_{\min}$) as midpoint. From the starting point of the new window formed, for each samples (say position k), 8-point average slope is computed at k and $(k + 25)$ position, to assess the position of upside and downside of positive R wave.

$$\text{Condition 1}:\ (\text{slope})_k\ > \ = \text{slp}_{\text{th}} \tag{2.14}$$

$$\text{Condition 2}:\ (\text{slope})_{k+25} < 0 \tag{2.15}$$

where $(\text{slope})_k$ is slope at k, and $(\text{slope})_{k+25}$ is the same at $k + 25$ position.

The STC (Eq. 2.14) will filter out any T peak being falsely detected, since QRS complex is always sharper than T wave. If Eq. (2.14) is satisfied, then Eq. (2.15) is searched to find a positive R peak. While both equations are satisfied at a sample position say k, it is concluded that a positive R peak exists. This is verified by a slope sign reversal within next 70-ms interval from current sample of reference k, confirming occurrence of an S peak. Hence, the correct position of R peak is determined by finding the index with highest amplitude within next 50 samples from k. For QS peaks (i.e., for negative QRS polarization), Eq. (2.14) will be only satisfied, but not Eq. (2.15) within current 96-ms window. In this case, it is concluded that a positive R peak does not exist and search for QS peak is initiated. The index with minimum amplitude within the current window of 96 ms is taken as the QS peak. Once the R peak (or QS peak) is determined, the next R-peak search is initiated at 400 samples upside the data array, assuming that the minimum R–R interval is 400 ms. If Eq. (2.14) is not satisfied throughout the entire 96-ms window formed around p_{max}

Table 2.5 S_e and P+ figures for Ptb-db using amplitude span detection

Patient file ID in Physionet	Lead I		Lead II		Lead aVR		Lead aVF		Lead V1		Lead V5	
	S_e	P+	S_e	P+	S_e	P+	S_e	P+	S_e	P+	S_e	P+
P237/s0465 (N)	100	100	100	100	100	100	100	100	100	100	100	100
P242/s0471 (N)	100	100	100	100	100	100	100	100	100	100	100	100
P248/s0481 (N)	100	100	100	100	100	100	100	100	100	100	100	100
P249/s0484 (M)	100	100	100	100	100	100	100	100	100	100	100	100
P267/s0504 (N)	100	100	100	100	100	100	100	100	100	100	100	100
P270/s0507 (Ant-Lat)	100	100	100	100	100	100	100	100	100	100	100	100
P269/s0508 (N)	100	100	100	100	100	100	100	100	100	100	100	100
P093/s0375(MI-Inf)	100	100	100	100	100	100	100	100	100	100	100	100
P093/s0378 (MI-Inf)	100	100	100	100	100	100	100	100	100	100	100	100
P002/0015 (MI-Ant)	100	100	100	100	100	100	100	100	100	100	100	100
P005/0021 (MI-Ant)	100	100	100	100	100	100	100	100	100	100	100	100
P001/0010 (Inf-Lat)	100	100	100	100	100	100	100	100	100	100	100	100

Narration N Normal; *MI* Myocardial infarction; *Ant* Anterio; *Inf* Inferio; *Lat* Latera; *M* Myocarditis

Table 2.6 S_e and P+ figures for mit-db using amplitude span detection

Patient file ID from Physionet with lead no.	R_e	P+
102 (v2)	100	100
103 (v2)	100	100
108 (v1)	96.15	100
109 (v1)	97.37	100
111 (v1)	100	100
114 (ML-II)	100	100
115 (v1)	100	100
123 (v5)	100	100
124 (v4)	100	100
201 (v1)	100	100

(or p_{min}), it is concluded that the amplitude threshold-based search might have captured a T wave. Hence, the next search is initiated from 200 samples downside along ECG array. The algorithm steps are given in the end of the chapter Appendix 3. Tables 2.5 and 2.6 represent some of the test results with ptb-db data and mit-db data, respectively. Figure 2.12a and b represent R-peak detection, baseline modulation correction using ptb-db and mit-db data, respectively.

2.4.2 Baseline Detection

The baseline point in each R–R interval is determined in the TP segment, which is the equipotential region between the T-offset point of current beat and P-onset point of following beat. For baseline point detection, a typical RR interval can be assumed to be consisting of two halves, with the left half containing T wave of the current beat and right half containing P wave of the following beat. The TP segment is nominally considered to be spanned between ±200 samples on either side of hypothetical mid-RR line. Since the algorithm is tested on noisy samples from Physionet, the average slope approach is used for minimizing abrupt fluctuations in the data. In the selected TP segment, baseline point is taken as the index with minimum absolute average slope over ±15 points. The baseline modulation is then applied to all samples between two successive baseline points by shifting them vertically up or down by an empirically determined formula, given in Eq. 2.16. The formula is based on the fact that a sample, positioned between two baseline points, which are vertically offset, is to be shifted in proportion to a fixed reference. To apply the correction throughout the dataset, this reference point is taken as first baseline point for the ECG dataset.

$$\partial_k = [x(k) - blp(i)] \times \frac{\Delta}{L} \tag{2.16}$$

where ∂_k is the vertical correction to be applied to a sample, $x(k)$, $blp(i)$ is the reference point, 'Δ' is the vertical offset, and 'L' is the index difference, respectively between two successive baseline points. The baseline correction is illustrated with the help of Fig. 2.13.

2.4.3 Determination of Fiducial Points

The detection of fiducial points from the ECG data is performed by a window search method, starting form the R peak of the respective cycle. For data analysis, we considered the following window sizes for different wave durations and intervals.

P wave: 100 ms
QRS: 120 ms
T wave: 160 ms
ST segment: 120 ms.

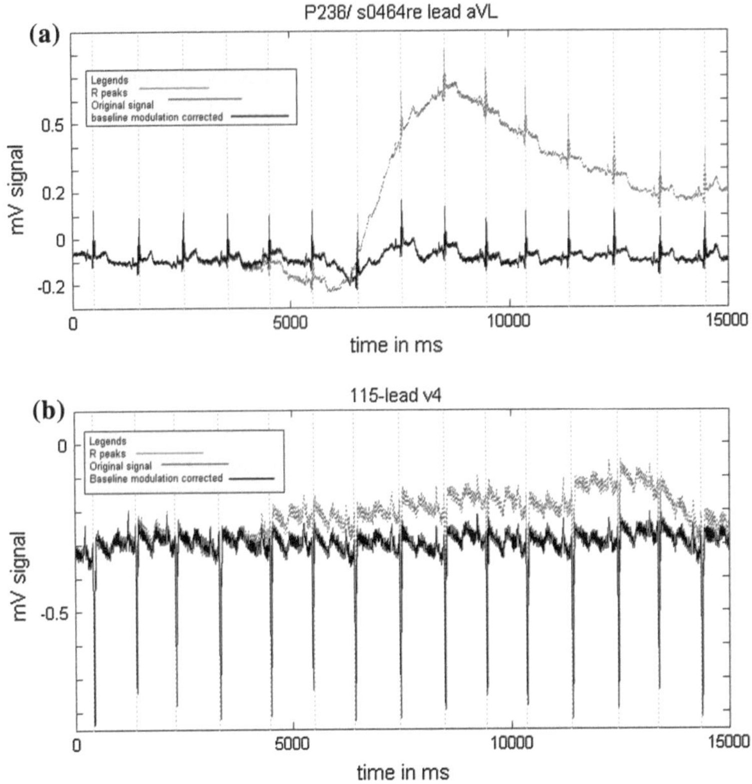

Fig. 2.12 R-peak detection from amplitude span detection. **a** using ptb-db data, **b** using mit-db data

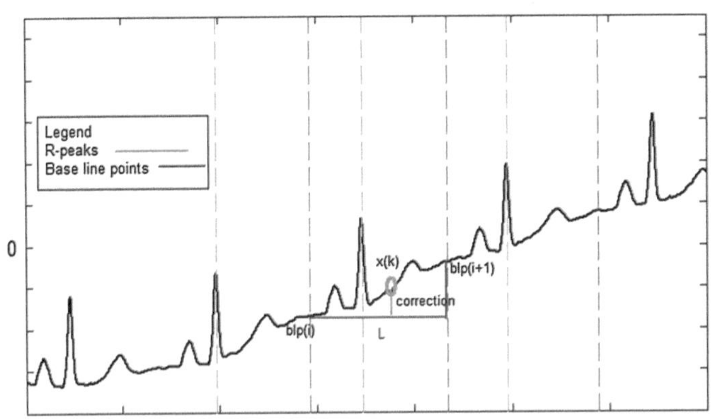

Fig. 2.13 Baseline modulation correction principle

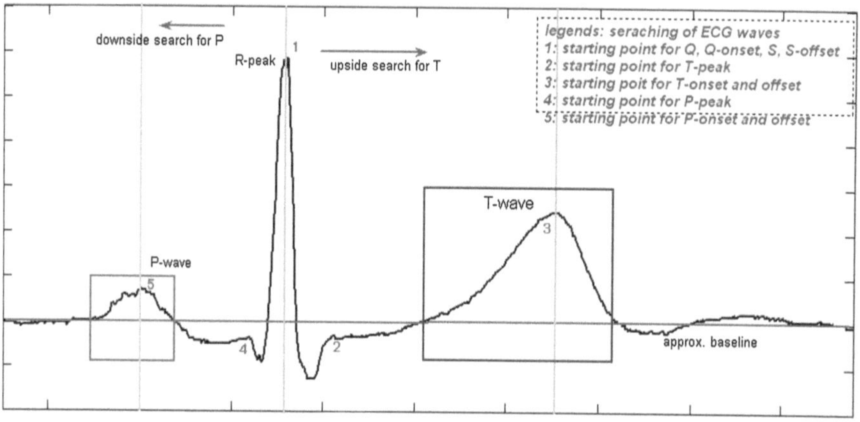

Fig. 2.14 Fiducial point detection in ECG wave

Figure 2.14 represents the starting points for search of different fiducial points. The following sections represent search criteria for different fiducial points.

2.4.3.1 Search for Q-peak and Q-onset Point:

The criteria for a valid Q peak are laid down as follows:

1. The voltage level should be equal or below the baseline voltage;
2. The magnitude of voltage should be lowest in a window of 50 ms downside from R peak;
3. There should be a slope sign reversal around of Q peak. This is ascertained by average slope computation at ±4-ms positions from Q peak.

If either condition is not satisfied, it is concluded that a valid Q peak does not exist and Q and Q-onset points coincide with each other. If a valid Q peak is found, the Q-offset point is determined by a window search of 50 ms downside of Q peak. The sample with minimum average slope within the window is considered as Q-onset. The algorithm steps are given in the end of the chapter Appendix 4.

2.4.3.2 Search for P, P-onset, and P-offset Point

The search is initiated from Q-onset point downside along the array to gradually reveal P, P-offset, and P-onset points. The curvature (positive or negate) of the P wave is determined by computing the 20-point average slope at 40 samples downside of Q-offset point. If the slope is found positive (negative), the P wave is positive (negative), and hence, it is found as the sample with highest (lowest) absolute magnitude with respect to baseline amplitude within a window of 70 samples downside the Q-onset.

The P-onset (P-offset) is found from the P peak by a window-based search along downside (upside). Both points are taken as the sample with minimum average slope computed over ±7 points on either side of P peak. The algorithm steps are given in the end of the chapter Appendix 5.

2.4.3.3 Search for S-peak and S-offset Point

The search is similar to finding Q and Q-onset, with the difference that it is initiated upside along the sample array starting from the R peak of the respective beat.

2.4.3.4 Search for T, T-onset, and T-offset Point

In principle, the search technique is similar to finding P, P-onset, and P-offset. At first, the T peak is found after determining its curvature, followed by T-onset and T-offset point detection. After determining all the characteristic points in the dataset, the following time-plane features are computed:

The characteristic points are detected in all beats over the dataset and the values of the different wave durations and intervals are computed. Figure 2.15 shows some qualitative results of accurate detection of characteristic points with 30,000 samples. For visual clarity, only few betas are shown. In the figure, the onset, offset, and wave peaks are indicated as separate colored lines along with the baseline index and baseline voltage. The determined and single baseline voltage is also shown as horizontal line. The following time-plane features are computed as follows;

QRS interval = S-offset index − Q-onset index
RR interval = R(i + 1) index − R(i) index
ST duration = T-onset index − S-offset index
QT duration = T-offset index − Q-onset index.

$$(\mathrm{QT})_c = \frac{(\mathrm{QT\ interval})}{\sqrt{\mathrm{R}} - \mathrm{R\ interval}}$$

P height = P-peak amplitude − Baseline voltage
T height = T-peak amplitude − Baseline voltage
QRS amplitude = R-peak amplitude − Q-peak amplitude
P-wave duration = P-offset-P-onset
T-wave duration = T-offset-T-onset

(a)
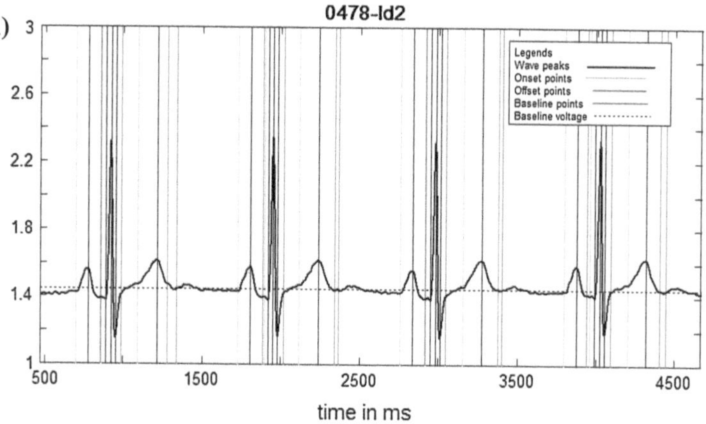

(b)
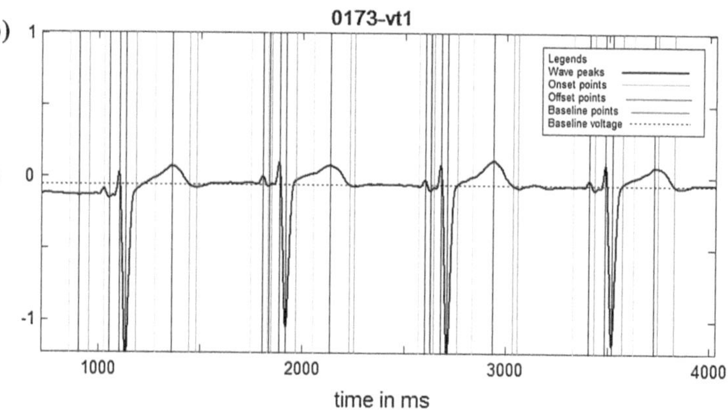

Fig. 2.15 Fiducial point determination from ptb-db data. **a** Normal data. **b** Abnormal data—MI-inferior

Variation among the different wave durations and intervals is computed and expressed as coefficient of variation (COV) figure, given as

$$C_v = \frac{\sigma}{\mu}$$

where σ is the standard deviation and μ is the mean value of the parameter. Table 2.7 shows some of the coefficients of variation figures of the time-plane signatures out of total 240 single-lead ptb-db data.

Table 2.7 Coefficient of variation figures (in 10^{-3})

Patient file ID in Physionet	Lead	Amplitude features			Wave interval features				
		QRS amplitude	T-height	P-height	RR	QRS	QT	P-width	T-width
P117/ s0292 (N)	II	0.734	0.225	0.412	0.963	0.099	0.145	0.252	0.096
	aVF	1.106	0.197	0.328	0.978	0.384	0.627	0.489	0.224
	V2	1.141	1.522	0.027	0.970	0.014	0.013	0.967	0.012
	V5	1.782	0.309	0.384	0.956	0.032	0.124	0.064	0.057
P105/ s0303(N)	II	7.626	6.475	0.155	1.329	0.245	4.726	0.105	1.798
	aVF	6.036	2.403	0.196	1.336	0.191	38.10	0.119	3.423
	V2	2.459	0.280	0.221	1.348	0.045	4.802	0.404	1.387
	V5	4.870	0.315	0.149	1.328	0.028	0.045	0.181	0.129
P246/ s0472(N)	II	10.76	7.269	1.294	0.064	0.191	34.83	0.065	0.622
	aVF	0.506	3.161	0.764	0.065	0.506	31.63	0.014	0.702
	V2	27.08	10.72	0.337	0.067	0.335	3.921	0.332	1.255
	V5	23.58	3.161	0.764	0.065	0.506	31.63	0.014	0.702
P266/ s0502(N)	II	0.865	0.157	0.045	0.075	0.222	0.144	0.045	0.159
	aVF	0.750	0.146	0.200	0.074	0.439	0.243	0.044	0.108
	V2	0.183	1.106	0.063	0.068	0.060	0.051	0.918	0.022
	V5	1.970	0.255	0.250	0.077	0.169	0.158	0.250	0.071
P277/ s0527(N)	II	1.002	0.058	0.257	3.199	0.083	0.173	0	0.052
	aVF	2.110	4.570	0.116	3.194	0.238	18.39	0.034	5.887
	V2	1.012	0.867	0.115	3.283	1.012	0.062	0.487	0.072
	V5	0.449	0.542	0.115	3.199	0.104	0.091	1.127	0
P093/ s0378 (MI – Inf)	II	29.67	0.817	24.00	0.515	0.015	55.60	0.198	0.600
	aVF	3.567	2.208	7.7259.588	1.854	0.053	12.45	0.730	1.301
	V3	0.664	2.546	0.291	0.543	0.180	0.209	0.507	0.013
	V5	1.146	2.987	0.081	0.529	0.053	0.068	0.267	0.118

(Narration: N: Normal; MI: Myocardial Infarction; Inf: Inferior)

The developed algorithm is tested with 240 single-lead ECG data from ptb-db database. Among the eight different features, the lowest COV is obtained with P-wave width with a value of 0.302×10^{-3} and highest with T-wave height, with a value of 7.87×10^{-3}. Considering all 12 leads in ptb-db files, an average value of 2.42×10^{-3} is obtained.

2.5 Conclusion

In this chapter, the basic techniques of computerized ECG analysis techniques are reviewed. R-peak detection is considered as one of the important criteria for accurate feature extraction. The performance evaluation parameters for R peak are also described. Algorithm steps for simple time-plane morphology-based feature extraction developed by us are elaborated in detail.

Acknowledgments Papers [26, 27], [36], [67], and [77] are the contribution from Biomedical Signal acquisition and Processing research group at Department of Applied Physics, University of Calcutta, India.

Appendix 1

R-peak Detection by Processing of Differential ECG Array

x = ECG data array
y = x(i + 1) − x(i) % D-ECG array
x_{max} = sample with maximum value on x-array
mx_slp = sample with maximum value on of y-array
r_th = R-threshold point index
slp_r = y (i-3: i+3); % rising edge 7-point average slope array
slp_f = y (i+30: i+36); % falling edge 7-point average slope array
aslp = abs (slp_r); % absolute values of slp_r
i = 1
% checking for criteria

1. if [(abs(x(i)) >= 0.5* x_{max})] & [(mean(slp_r) > 0) & (mean(slp_f) < 0)] & [mean(aslp) >= 0.30*mx_slp), then
   (a) r_th(k) = i; % possible R-threshold point
   (b) k = k+1; i = i+300;
   (c) go to step 3
2. else i = i+1;
3. if end of data array y, skip step 4
4. go to step 1
5. for each r_th index value k1, find out local maxima or minima on k1 to k1+50-ms window

   n = number of total R-threshold points

   (i) k1 = 1; i = r_th(k1); k = 1; $x1_{max}$ = x(i); $x1_{min}$ = x(i) % initialization
   (ii) if x(i) < $x1_{max}$ skip step (iii)
   (iii) $x1_{max}$ = x(i); r1 = i;
   (iv) if x(i) > $x1_{min}$ skip step (v)
   (v) $x1_{min}$ = x(i); r2 = i
   (vi) i = i +1;
   (vii) if i = r_th(k1) + 50 go to step (ix)
   (viii) go to step (ii)
   (ix) if slp_f(i + 15) < 0 skip step (x) % checking for slope reversal
   (x) r_pk (k) = r2, k = k + 1; go to step (xii) % taking local minima as R peak
   (xi) r_pk (k) = r2, k = k + 1, % taking local maxima as R peak

(xii) if k1 < n, skip step (xiii)
(xiii) stop
(xiv) i = r_th(k1 + 1), go to step (i) for next search

Appendix 2

R-peak Detection by Squared Derivative ECG Array

i = data array index;
y = lead data array;

1. Spline smoothing operation on samples with a tolerance of .002, resulting array y2
2. y1(i) = y2(i)* y2(i) %Squaring of array y2

   % Lagrange's five-point interpolation for derivative

3. d1(i + 2) = [y1(i)-(8*y1(i + 1)) + (8*y1(i + 3))-(y1(i + 4))]/(12*0.002);
4. d1′(i) = d1(i) * d1(i); %Squaring of array d1

   % Lagrange's five-point interpolation for derivative

5. d2 = [d1′(i)-(8*d1′(i + 1)) + (8*d1′(i + 3))-(d1′(i + 4))]/(12*0.002);
6. d2′(i) = d2(i)*d2(i); %Squaring of array d2
7. find out maximum value in d2′ array, say this is $d2_{max}$
8. find out the positions in array d2′ with amplitudes greater than $0.05*d2_{max}$ say this array is i3.

   (i) i = 1; k1 = 1;
   (ii) if d2′(i) < 0.05* $d2_{max}$, go to step (v)
   (iii) i = i + 1; go to step (ii)
   (iv) if end of data array d2′, go to step 9
   (v) i3(k1) = i; k1 = k1 + 1; i = i + 1; go to step (ii)

9. for each i3 index (k), find out maximum y2 amplitude in the neighbor of 90-ms window

   (i) j = i3(k); k1 = 1
   (ii) r = R-peak index array
   (iii) $y2_{max}$ = y2(j − 48);
   (iv) if y2(j − 45) < y2(j) skip step (v)
   (v) $y2_{max}$ = y2(j − 48); r1 = j − 45;
   (vi) j = j + 1;
   (vii) if j < i3(k) + 48 go to step (iv)

Appendix 3

R-peak Detection by Amplitude Span Detection of QRS

1. g_span = 0; mx_slp = 0; i = 1; mx_val = x(i), mn_val = x(i) % initialization
2. window formation of 96 ms
3. calculate 8-point average slope, av_slp
4. if av_slp < mx_slp, skip step 5
5. mx_slp = av_slp
6. span = (mx_val − mn_val) %calculate amplitude span
7. if span < g_span, skip step 8
8. span = g_span
9. slide window by 20 ms
10. if end of data array, skip step 11
11. go to step 2
12. $span_{th}$ = 0.8*g_span; slp_{th} = 0.8*mx_slp, again start from beginning of data array
13. calculate span over 96 ms
14. if span > = $span_{th}$, go to step 17
15. slide window by 20 ms
16. go to step 13
17. calculate 16-point average slope on upside and downside slope with respect to maximum and minimum points p_{max} and p_{min}
18. if (slp_r_{20-} > 0) & (slp_r_{18+} < 0) go to step 23
19. if (slp_q_{20-} < 0) & (slp_q_{18+} > 0) skip step 20
20. slide window by 20 ms, go to step 13
21. shift window with respect to p_{min} as midpoint, start from beginning of this window
22. go to step 24
23. Shift window with respect to p_{max} as midpoint, start from beginning of this window
24. calculate av_slp_i and av_slp_{i+25}
25. if av_slp_i < 0.8*mx_slp go to step 29
26. if av_slp_{i+25} < 0, go to step 31
27. if window end arrived, go to step 33
28. i = i + 1, go to step 26
29. if window end arrived, i = i + 200, go to step 13
30. i = i+1, go to step 24
31. find local maximum (say i_{max}) i to i + 50, r_pk = i_{max}
32. i = i + 400; go to step 35
33. find local minimum (say, i_{min}) at i to i-50, r_pk = i_{min}
34. i = i + 400; go to step 35

35. if end of array skip step 36
36. go to step 13 for next search
37. stop

Appendix 4

The algorithm steps for Q and Q-onset:
i = ECG data array index; y = magnitude; y(blp) = baseline voltage;
slp(i) = 8-point average slope; slp_mn = minimum average slope
k1 = 1; % R-peak index

1. i = r(k1) % R-peak index
2. if y(i) ≤ y(blp) go to step 6% baseline cross
3. i = i-1
4. if i = r(k1)-50 go to step 11% no defined Q peak exits
5. go to step 2
6. k = i
7. if (slp(i+4) > 0) & (slp(i-4) < 0) go to step 11
8. i = k-1;
9. if i = k-30 go to step 13
10. go to step 7
11. k = Q_indx(k1); % Q peak obtained
12. go to step 14 for Q-onset detection
13. consider Q peak as slope with minimum average slope in R to R-50 zone

    (i) i = r(k1)
    (ii) slp_mn = abs[slp(i)]; % initialization
    (iii) if abs[slp(i)] ≥ slp_mn skip step (iv)
    (iv) slp_mn = slp(i); indx = i
    (v) i = i-1;
    (vi) if i = r(k1)-50 skip step (vii)
    (vii) i = i-1; go to step (iii)
    (viii) Q_indx(k1) = indx; % accept index with absolute minimum slope
    (ix) Qon_indx(k1) = indx;
    (x) go to step 22

14. k2 = Q_indx(k1)
15. slp_mn = abs[slp(k2)]; % initialization
16. if abs[slp(k2)] > slp_mn skip step 17
17. slp_mn = slp(k2); indx = k2
18. k2 = k2-1;
19. if i = r(k1)-50 skip step 20
20. i = i-1; go to step 16

21. Qon_indx(k1) = indx;
22. k1 = k1 + 1;
23. if end of R-peak array index is arrived, skip step 24
24. go to step 2 for next Q-peak and Q_onset detection
25. stop

Appendix 5

The algorithms steps for P, P-onset:
y(blp) = baseline voltage
k = 1% Q-onset array index
slp(i) = 15-point average slope computed at index i

1. i = Q_on(k) − 40% initialization
2. if slp(i) > 0, go to step 11% inverted P wave
3. i = Q_on(k)
4. y_{max} = y(i) − y(blp)
5. if y(i) − y(blp) < y_{max} skip step 6
6. y_{max} = y(i) − y(blp), indx = i;
7. i = i − 1;
8. if i < Q_on(k) − 50, skip step 9
9. P(k) = indx, go to step 19% P-wave peak
10. go to step 5
11. i = Q_on(k)
12. y_{min} = y(i) − y(blp)
13. if y(i) − y(blp) > $y_{min,}$ skip step 14
14. y_{min} = y(i) − y(blp); indx = i;
15. i = i − 1
16. if i < Q_on(k) -50, skip step 17
17. P(k) = indx % P-wave peak
18. go to step 13

% P-onset determination

19. i = P(k), slp_mn = abs[slp(i)] % initialization
20. slp_mn = abs[slp(i)] % initialization of minimum average slope
21. if abs[slp (i)] ≤ slp_mn, skip step 22
22. slp_mn = abs[slp(i)], indx = i;
23. i = i − 1;
24. if i > P(k) − 70 skip step 25
25. P_on(k) = indx, go to step 27
26. go to step 21

% P-offset determination

27. i = P(k); slp_mn = abs[slp(i)] % initialization
28. slp_mn = abs[slp(i)] % initialization of minimum average slope
29. if slp (i) > slp_mn, skip step 30
30. slp_mn = abs[slp(i)], indx = i;
31. i = i + 1;
32. if i < P(k) + 70 skip step 33
33. P_off(k) = indx,
34. k = k + 1
35. go to step 1 for next P-wave detection

References

1. Rangyyan RM. Biomedical signal anal: a case study approach. Singapore: Wiley; 2002.
2. Huhta JC, Webster JG. 60-Hz interference in electrocardiography. IEEE Tran in Biomed Eng BME-20. 1973;2:91–101.
3. Webster JG. Reducing motion artifacts and interference in biopotentials recording. IEEE tran in Biomed Eng BME-31. 1984;12:823–826.
4. Narwaria RP, Verma S, Singhal PK. Removal of baseline wander and power line interference from ECG signal—a survey approach. Int J Electron Eng. 2011;3(1):107–11.
5. Hirano K, Nishimura S, Mitra SK. Design of digital notch filters. IEEE Tran on Comm COM-22. 1974;7:964–974.
6. Bailey JJ, Berson AS, Garson A, Horan LG, Macfarlane PW, Mortara DW, Zywietz C. Recommendations for standardization and specifications in automated electrocardiography: Bandwidth and digital signal processing. A report for health professionals by ad hoc writing group of the committee on electrocardiography and cardiac electrophysiology of the council on clinical cardiology, American heart association. Circulation. 1990;81:730.
7. Thakor NV, Moreau D. Design and analysis of quantized coefficient digital filters: application to biomedical signal processing with microprocessors. Med biol Eng Comput. 1987;25(1):18–25.
8. Hamilton PS. A comparison of adaptive and nonadaptive filters for reduction of power line interference in the ECG. IEEE Tran on Biomed Eng. 1996;43(1):105–9.
9. Ahlstrom ML, Tompkins WJ. Digital filters for real-time ECG signal processing using microprocessors. IEEE Tran on Biomed Eng BME-32. 1985;9:708–713.
10. Pei SC, Tseng CC. Elimination of AC interference in electrocardiogram using IIR notch filter with transient suppression. IEEE Tran Biomed Eng. 1995;42(11):1128–32.
11. Ider YZ, Koyemen H. A new technique for line interference monitoring and reduction in biopotential amplifiers. IEEE Tran Biomed Eng. 1990;37(6):624–31.
12. van Alste JA, Schilder TS. Removal of base-line wander and power-line interference from the ECG by an efficient FIR filter with a reduced number of taps. IEEE Tran Biomed Eng BME-32. 1985;12:1052–1060.
13. Thakor NV, Zhu YS. Applications of adaptive filtering to ECG analysis: noise cancellation and arrhythmia detection. IEEE Tran Biomed Eng. 1991;38(8):785–794.
14. Jane R, Laguna P, Thakor NV, Caminal P. Adaptive baseline wander removal in the ECG: comparative analysis with cubic spline technique. In: Proceedings of computers in cardiology, 1992, 11–14 Oct 1992, pp 143–146.
15. Meyera CR, Keiser HN. Electrocardiogram baseline noise estimation and removal using cubic splines and state-space computation techniques. Comput Biomed Res. 1977;10(5):459–70.

16. Shusterman V, Shah SI, Beigel A, Anderson KP. Enhancing the precision of ECG baseline correction: selective filtering and removal of residual error. Comput Biomed Res. 2000;33(2):144–60.
17. Almenar V, Albiol A. A new adaptive scheme for ECG enhancement. Signal Process. 1999;75(3):253–63.
18. Sun Y, Chan KL, Krishnan SM. ECG signal conditioning by morphological filtering. Comput Biol Med. 2002;32(6):465–479.
19. Widrow B, Glover JR, McCool JM, Kaunitz J, Williams CS, Hearn RH, Zeidler JR, Dong E, Goodlin RC. Adaptive noise canceling: principles and applications. Proc IEEE. 1975;63(12):1692–716.
20. Mneimneh MA, Yaz EE, Johnson MT, Povinelli RJ. An adaptive kalman filter for removing baseline wandering in ECG signals. In: Proceeding of Computers in cardiology, 2006, 17–20 Sep, pp 253–256.
21. Romero I. PCA and ICA applied to noise reduction in multi-lead ECG. In: Proceedings of computing in cardiology, 2011;38, 18–21 Sep 2011 pp. 613–616.
22. Chawla MPS. PCA and ICA processing methods for removal of artifacts and noise in electrocardiograms: a survey and comparison. Appl Soft Comput. 2011;11(2):2216–2226.
23. Kotas M. Application of projection pursuit based robust principal component analysis to ECG enhancement. Biomed Signal Process Control. 2006;1(4):289–98.
24. Farahabadi E, Farahabadi A, Rabbani H, Mahjoob MP, Dehnavi AM. Noise removal from electrocardiogram signal employing an artificial neural network in wavelet domain. In: Proceedings of the 9th international conference on information technology and applications in biomedicine (ITAB),2009, 5–7Nov 2009, pp. 1–4.
25. Sotos JM, Arnau JMB, Aranda AMT, Melendez CS. Removal of muscular and artefacts noise from the ECG by a neural network. In: Proceedings of 5th IEEE international conference on industrial informatics, 2007, 23–25 June 2007, pp. 687–692.
26. Pal S, Mitra M. Detection of ECG characteristic points using multiresolution wavelet analysis based selective coefficient method. Measurement. 2010;43(2):255–61.
27. Banerjee S, Gupta R, Mitra M. Delineation of ECG characteristic features using multiresolution wavelet analysis method. Measurement. 2012;45(3):474–87.
28. Tikkanen PE. Nonlinear wavelet and wavelet packet denoising of electrocardiogram signal. Biol Cybern. 1999;80(4):259–67.
29. Donoho DL. Denoising by soft-thresholding. IEEE Tran Inf Theory. 1995;41(3):613–627.
30. Donoho DL, Johnstone LM. Ideal spatial adaptation by spatial shrinkage. Biometrika. 1994;425–455.
31. Cherkassky V, Kilts S. Myopotential denoising of ECG signals using wavelet thresholding methods. Neural Netw. 2001;14(8):1129–37.
32. Kania M, Fereniec M, Maniewski R. Wavelet denoising for multi-lead high resolution ECG signals. Meas Sci Rev. 2007;7(2, 4):30–33.
33. Kirst M, Glauner B, Ottenbacher J. Using DWT for ECG motion artifact reduction with noise-correlating signals. In: Proceedings of 33rd annual international conference of the IEEE EMBS Boston, 2011, 30 Aug–3 Sep, pp. 4804-4807.
34. Chmelka L, Kozumplík J. Wavelet-based wiener filter for electrocardiogram signal denoising. In: Proceedings of computers in cardiology, 2005, 25–28 Sep 2005, pp. 771–774.
35. Velasco MB, Weng B, Barner KE. ECG signal denoising and baseline wander correction based on the empirical mode decomposition. Comput Biol Med. 2008;38(1):1–13.
36. Pal S, Mitra M. Empirical mode decomposition based ECG enhancement and QRS detection. Comput Biol Med. 2012;42(1):83–92.
37. Kotas M. Robust projective filtering of time-warped ECG beats. Comput Methods Prog Biomed. 2008;92(2):161–72.
38. Goldberger JG, Jason Ng, editors. Practical signal and image processing in clinical cardiography. USA: Springer; 2010. p. 43.
39. Kohler BU, Henning C, Orglmeister R. The principles of software QRS detection IEEE Eng Medicine Biol Magazine. 2002;21(1):42–57, Jan–Feb 2002.

40. Holsinger WP, Kempner KM, Miller MH. A QRS preprocessor based on digital differentiation. IEEE Tran Biomed Eng BME-18. 1971;3:212–217.
41. Ahlstrom ML, Tompkins WJ. Automated high-speed analysis of Holter tapes with microcomputers. IEEE Trans Biomed Eng. 1983;30:651–7.
42. Okada M. A digital filter for the QRS complex detection. IEEE Tran Biomed Eng BME-26. 1979;12:700–703.
43. Ligtenburg A, Kunt M. A robust-digital QRS detection algorithm for arrhythmia monitoring. Comput Biomed Res. 1983;16(3):273–86.
44. Pan J, Tompkins WJ. A real time QRS detection algorithm. IEEE Tran Biomed Eng BME-32. 1985;3:230–236.
45. Hamilton PS, Tompkins WJ. Quantitative investigation of QRS detection rules using the MIT/BIH arrhythmia database IEEE Tran Biomed Eng BME-33. 1986;12:1157–1165.
46. Azreno NM, Deng ZD, Poon CS. Analysis of first-derivative based QRS detection algorithms. IEEE Tran Biomed Eng. 2008;55(2):478–84.
47. Borjesson PO, Pahlm O, Sörnmo L, Nygards ME. Adaptive QRS detection based on maximum a posteriori estimation. IEEE Tran Biomed Eng BME-29. 1982;5:341–351.
48. Sörnmo L, Pahlm O, Nygards ME. Adaptive QRS detection: a study of performance. IEEE Tran Biomed Eng BME-32. 1985;6:392–401.
49. Trahanias PE. An approach to QRS detection using mathematical morphology. IEEE Tran Biome Eng. 1993;40(2):201–5.
50. Ghaffari A, Golbayani H, Ghasemi M. A new mathematical based QRS detector using continuous wavelet transform. Comput Elect Eng. 2008;34(2):81–91.
51. Islam Md S, Alajlan N. A morphology alignment method for resampled heartbeat signals. Biomed Signal Proc Control. 2013;8(3):315–24.
52. Suppappola S, Sun Y. Nonlinear transforms of ECG signals for digital QRS detection: a quantitative analysis. IEEE Tran Biome Eng. 1994;41(4):397–400.
53. Benitez D, Gaydecki PA, Zaidi A, Fitzpatrick AP. The use of Hilbert transform for ECG signal analysis. Comput Biol Med. 2001;31(5):399–406.
54. Benitez DS, Gaydecki PA, Zaidi A, Fitzpatrick AP. A new QRS detection algorithm based on the Hilbert transform. In: Proceedings of computers in cardiology, 2000, 24–27 Sep 2000, pp. 379–382.
55. Kadambe S, Murray R, Bartels GB. Wavelet transform-based QRS complex detector. IEEE Tran Biome Eng. 1999;46(7):838–48.
56. Zhang F, Lian Y. Novel QRS detection by CWT for ECG sensor. In: Proceedings of IEEE biomedical circuits and systems conference (BIOCAS), 2007, 27–30 Nov. 2007, pp. 211–214.
57. Bahoura M, Hassani M, Hubin M. DSP implementation of wavelet transform for real time ECC wave forms detection and heart rate analysis. Comput methods Prog Biomed. 1997;52(1):35–44.
58. Zhu K, Noakes PD, Green ADP. ECG monitoring with artificial neural networks. In: Proceedings of 2nd international conference on artificial neural networks, 1991, 18–20 Nov 1991, Colchester, pp. 205–209.
59. Xue Q, Hue YH, Tompkins WJ. Neural-network-based adaptive matched filtering for QRS detection. IEEE Tran Biomed Eng. 1992;39(4):317–29.
60. Behrad A, Faez K. New method for QRS-wave recognition in ECG using MART neural network. In: Proceedings of the 7th Australian and New Zealand intelligent information systems conference, 2001, 18–21 Nov 2001, pp. 291–296.
61. Poli R, Cagnoni S, Valli G. Genetic design of optimum linear and nonlinear QRS detectors. IEEE Tran Biomed Eng. 1995;42(11):1137–1141.
62. Karpagachelvi S, Arthanari M, Sivakumar M. ECG feature extraction techniques-a survey approach. Int J Comput Sci Inf Secur. 2010;8(1):76–80.
63. Vaneghi FM, Oladazimi M, Shiman F, Kordi A, Safari MJ, Ibrahim F. A comparative approach to ECG feature extraction methods. In: Proceedings of 3rd international conference on intelligent systems modeling and simulation, 2012,08–10 Feb, Malaysia, pp. 252–256.

64. Milliken JA, Wartak J, Skoulikidis AP, Lywood DW. Use of computers in the interpretations of electrocardiograms. Can Med Assoc J. 1969;101(7):39–43.
65. Murray TH. The design, development, and implementation of a microprocessor-based ECG analysis system. Behav Res Methods Instrum. 1982;14(2):281–9.
66. Mazomenos EB, Chen T, Acharyya A, Bhattacharya A, Rosengarten J, Maharatna K. A time-domain morphology and gradient based algorithm for ECG feature extraction. In: Proceedings of IEEE international conference on industrial technology (ICIT), 2012, 19–21 March 2012, pp. 117–122.
67. Chatterjee HK, Gupta R, Mitra M. A statistical approach for determination of time plane features from digitized ECG. Comput Biol Med. 2011;41(5):278–84.
68. Olivas ES, Sober MM, Maravilla JC, Guerrero-Mart′ınez JF, Gasco JC, Lopez JE. Application of adaptive signal processing for determining the limits of P and T waves in an ECG. IEEE Tran Biomed Eng. 1998;45(8):1077–80.
69. Chazal P, O'Dwyer M, Reilly RB. Automatic classification of heart beats using ECG morphology and heart beat interval features. IEEE Tran Biomed Eng. 2004;51(7):1196–206.
70. Chazal P, Reilly RB. A patient- adapting heart beat classifier using ECG morphology and heartbeat interval features. IEEE Tran Biomed Eng. 2006;53(12):2535–43.
71. Tadejko P, Rakowski W. Mathematical morphology based ECG feature extraction for the purpose of heart beat classification. In: Proceedings of 6th international conference on computer information systems and industrial management applications (CISIM), 2007, 28–30 June 2007, Poland, pp. 322–327.
72. Li C, Zheng C, Tai C. Detection of ECG characteristic points using wavelet transform. IEEE Tran Biomed Eng. 1995;42(1):21–8.
73. Saxena SC, Kumar V, Hamde ST. Feature extraction from ECG signals using wavelet transforms for disease diagnosis. Int J Syst Sci. 2003;33(13):1073–85.
74. Martinez JP, Almeida R, Olmos S, Rocha AP, Laguna P. A wavelet-based ECG delineation: evaluation of standard databases. IEEE Tran Biomed Eng. 2004;51(4):570–81.
75. Sahambi JS, Tendon SN, Bhatt RKP. Using wavelet transforms for ECG characterization an online digital processing system. IEEE Eng Med Biol Mag. 1997;16(1):77–83.
76. Benitez D, Gaydecki PA, Zaidi A, Fitzpatrick AP. The use of the Hilbert transform in ECG signal analysis. Comput Biol Med. 2001;31:399–406.
77. Mukhopadhyay SK, Mitra M, Mitra S. ECG feature extraction using differentiation, Hilbert transform and slope reversal approach. J Med Eng Tech. 2012;36(7):372–86.
78. Martis RJ, Chakraborty C, Roy AK. An integrated ECG feature extraction scheme using PCA and wavelet transform. In: Proceedings of annual IEEE India conference (INDICON), 2009, 18–20 Dec, Gujarat, pp. 1–4.
79. Lee GG, Hu JY, Chen CF, Lin HH. Gabor feature extraction for electrocardiogram signals. In: Proceedings of IEEE biomedical circuits and systems conference (BioCAS), 2012, 28–30 Nov, Taiwan, pp. 304–307.
80. Ghongade R, Ghatol AA. Performance analysis of feature extraction schemes for artificial neural network based ECG classification. In: Proceedings of international conference on computational intelligence and multimedia applications, 2007, 13–15 Dec 2007, Tamilnadu, pp. 486–490.
81. Hildebrand FB (1974) Introduction to Numerical Analysis, 2nd Edition, Tata McGraw-Hill Publishing Company Ltd., New Delhi.

Chapter 3
ECG Acquisition in a Computer

3.1 Introduction

Most of the modern electrocardiogram recording systems in a clinical setup use a desktop computer as the final data acquisition element. This allows each storage and retrieval of records and data sharing with concerned medical experts on demand. Perhaps the most advantageous feature of computerized acquisition is ECG analysis for feature extraction using software. Presently, a few standard ECG analysis softwares are available which provide accurate preliminary level features for the cardiologists for 'assisted diagnoses.' Often, they include a powerful 'visualization tool' that felicitates detailed investigation using the ECG plot on the computer screen. The objective of this chapter is to highlight the block structure and key functional features of a typical ECG acquisition system in desktop computer. This is followed by a description of a PC-based single-channel ECG acquisition system using serial port communication.

3.2 ECG Acquisition in a Clinical Setup

Electrocardiograph still remains the most common cardiac investigation device in the primary care clinics all over the world. This huge popularity is primarily due to its non-invasive, painless nature to the patient, and easy procedural steps.

Most common form of ECG tests is 'routine test,' classified as per the ways the tests are performed as follows:

1. Rest ECG examination—patient lies in rest and multilead recording is done.
2. Exercise ECG—it is also called 'stress ECG' or 'treadmill test' (TMT), and the patient is required to exercise in a treadmill machine.
3. Holter test—this is a prolonged recording (24 or 48 h) where the patient can lead his normal life.

R. Gupta et al., *ECG Acquisition and Automated Remote Processing*,
DOI: 10.1007/978-81-322-1557-8_3, © Springer India 2014

4. Spatial recording—it is also called vectorcardiography, which is performed on 3 orthogonal leads.
5. Heart mapping—it is also called surface ECG test, which employs multiple channel (as many as 80 leads) recording by placing electrodes on heart muscles.

Conventional ECG recording generates traces of 12 leads (3 bipolar standard leads, 3 augmented limb leads, and 6 chest leads) in a chart recorder, printing 5–6 beats (R–R intervals) per lead for visual examination by a cardiologist. The lead recordings may be sequential, i.e., the medical professional selects the leads to be traced by switch positions on the recorder or, simultaneous, where recording of all 12-leads are traced.

Mechanical-type recording systems employ a current activated stylus, which produces an impression on a thermally sensitive paper moving at 25 mm/s. The inertia of the mechanical system puts an upper limit of recoding at 80 Hz. Since the clinical bandwidth of ECG is in the range 0.05–130 Hz, personal computer-based systems are gradually replacing mechanical recorders. Following, presently many ECG recorders provide a port for connectivity to a computer for direct acquisition of ECG samples. Further details of electrocardiography can be found in [1–3].

3.3 ECG Acquisition Systems

3.3.1 ECG Signal Characteristics and Artifacts

In this section, we describe the basic electrical characteristics of ECG signal which are essential for design and development of a hardware acquisition module for its collection from a patient. ECG is a low-amplitude (± 3 mV maximum) and non-stationery signal. Most of the clinically significant information in ECG is found in the spectral band 0–100 Hz.

Even with utmost care during the record, the ECG signal is contaminated with several types of unwanted signals, collectively called 'artifacts.' Some of these are of physiological origin, i.e., generated within human body and the others non-physiological, i.e., external to the body. Some of these signals have overlapping spectral band with the ECG signal itself, which means designing a simple band-pass filter is not sufficient for their elimination. The sources of artifacts are as follows:

1. **Electromyography (EMG) noise**: Picked up due to muscular activity of the patient. Their amplitude and frequency band, 0.1–1 mV and 5 Hz–1 kHz, respectively, are partly overlapping with ECG signal. EMG noise, if not properly taken care off, may completely destroy the signal based analysis. For short-duration clinical testing, the patient is advised to lie on resting condition so as to minimize the noise. However, for long-term Holter monitoring, this EMG noise is unavoidable.

2. **Power Line interference (PLI)**: These are picked up on the lead wires of neighboring power line cables, due to capacitive coupling with ECG lead wires. So, a 50/60 ± 0.2 Hz current flows through the lead wires to ground through the patient body. Sometimes, the equivalent voltage drop that appears as a common-mode signal to the input of the ECG amplifier can be as high as 20 mV, which is four times greater than the maximum ECG amplitude itself. A detailed discussion on PLI is given in [4]. A measurement technique of power line interference technique is described in [5]. In another approach [6], line interference reduction is described where the line reference signal is simultaneously measured and a scaled version is subtracted from the ECG by signal averaging.
3. **Electrode pop or contact noise**: Sometimes loss of contact between the patient skin and electrode may cause a temporary saturation of the amplifier output for certain period of time.
4. **Baseline wander**: This is due to respiration of the patient during ECG. The lung volume change during the respiration process changes the impedance between the heart muscle and electrode. This causes baseline (isoelectric level segments) of the ECG to oscillate at a very-low-frequency drifting between 0.15 and 0.3 Hz.
5. **Motion Artifacts**: Due to improper 'preparation' of the skin, or patient movement, a slow movement of the electrodes may occur in long-term recording using wearable sensors. Motion artifact has a significant overlap with ECG signal spectrum in the range 1–10 Hz. This results in an abrupt baseline jump or complete saturation of amplifier output for 0.5 s.
6. **Electrosurgical noise**: This is the noise generated by neighboring medical equipments in the clinical setup at frequencies between 100 kHz and 1 MHz.
7. **Amplifier noise**: Noise and drift are two unwanted signals that are generated within the amplifier that contaminate a biopotential signal under measurement. 'Noise' generally refers to undesirable signals with spectral components above 0.1 Hz, while 'drift' generally refers to slow changes in the baseline at frequencies below 0.1 Hz. The noise and drift are measured either in microvolts peak to peak ($\mu V_{p\text{-}p}$) or in microvolts root mean square (RMS) (μV_{RMS}) and appear as if they were applied as differential input voltage.
8. **Quantization noise**: The AD converter, having a finite bit width, samples the amplified ECG to generate a sequence of discrete data, which are digitized representations approximated to the nearest bit. Quantization noise thus refers to this truncation of the analog samples, which are of infinite resolution, to a binary number of finite width and equal to ±1 LSB of the AD converter.

A detailed discussion on ECG artifacts can be found in [7–8]. These artifacts can be minimized by suitable designs and clinical setup; however, it is impossible to completely eliminate those altogether using hardware designs. Nowadays, many soft computational techniques are available which are used for denoising digitized ECG.

3.3.2 Functional Blocks of a Digital ECG Acquisition System

The generalized block diagram of a digital ECG acquisition hardware module is shown in Fig. 3.1. It can be divided into three functional blocks connected in sequence, viz., analog front end, AD conversion, and a processor with a bus interface capability. The function of the analog front end is to reject (or at least minimize) the artifacts associated with the biosignal at the input, amplify the biosignal to the input span of the AD converter, and maintain galvanic isolation of the patient from power line or any accidental transient voltage surge.

The first stage of the analog front end is patient isolation circuit, which prevents any current from the acquisition circuit to flow through the patient body. The first stage provides low offset, high CMRR instrumentation amplifier (INA). This is the most important of the circuit since it determines the quality of the acquired signal. The next stage is a low pass filter and a notch filter to block high frequency and power line interference. If the AD converter is operated in unipolar mode of operation, then a level shifter is included at the final stage of analog conditioning. The output from this stage is 0–5 V. Today's ECG acquisition cards employ a 12- or 16-bit AD converter, which supplies the quantized samples to the high-end microcontroller. The microcontroller provides some intelligent features to the acquisition module like self-test, auto-calibration. However, its main function is to deliver the data samples to the bus interface unit for delivery to the final storage device, which may be a computer, personal digital assistant, mobile phone, iPad, etc. For this, the microcontroller is provided with a small buffer memory and associated peripherals. A graphical front end at the acquisition device may provide some flexibility in selecting the sampling rate, duration of acquisition, etc.

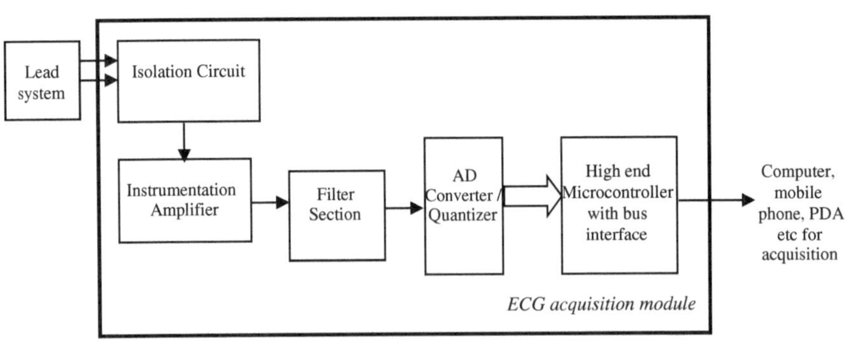

Fig. 3.1 Block diagram of a digital ECG acquisition module

3.3.3 ECG Amplifier and their Design Enhancements

The first block of the analog front end is essentially an AC-coupled low-offset high-CMRR INA. The desirable characteristics of an ECG amplifier are given [9] as

1. **Gain**: The gain of a biopotential amplifier (BPA) is expressed in decibels as

$$\text{gain (dB)} = 20\log_{10}(\text{linear gain}) \tag{3.1}$$

The nominal gain of ECG amplifier is around 750.

2. **Bandwidth**: The frequency bandwidth of the amplifier should be designed so as to amplify, without attenuation, all frequency components of the ECG.
3. **Common-mode rejection (CMR)**: Some of the artifacts picked up from external sources appear as 'common-mode signal' (i.e., at both input leads) at the input of the amplifier. Thus, CMR of the BPA qualitatively describes its capability to reject these low-amplitude signals at the input stage and is measured by common-mode rejection ratio (CMRR), which is defined as

$$\text{CMRR (dB)} = 20\ \log_{10}\left(\frac{A_d}{A_{\text{cm}}}\right) \tag{3.2}$$

where A_{cm} stands for gain from common-mode input and A_d stands for gain from differential input. The effect of common-mode impedance unbalance and electrode–skin impedance on CMRR is analyzed in [10] using four-terminal method. In [11], a novel, balanced, AC-coupled, differential amplifier with AC-coupled input stage and a third stage providing ground path using a third (common) electrode is described. The CMRR of ECG amplifier greatly depends on matching of the resistance pairs in the INA block, which in practical circuits is difficult to achieve. This results in an amplification of the DC offset voltage, mainly caused due to electrode–skin impedance and PLI. In [12], a design approach is proposed, which does not rely on matching of resistors. It includes a fully differential DC suppression circuit in addition to AC coupling for full restoration of DC biopotential signals. The power line frequency (and its harmonics) induces stray capacitive coupling with the patient body and lead wires. The order of these capacitances is 60 pfd, which corresponds to an impedance of 64 kΩ at 50 Hz. The leakage current produces a voltage drop w.r.t. ground, which appears as common-mode signal to the first stage of the ECG amplifier. To minimize this interference effect, the CMR plays a vital role in rejecting this noise. The typical CMRR of around 1,000 can help to minimize the interference.
4. **Recovery**: Sudden movement of the patient during ECG procedure can saturate the amplifier output due to high-amplitude input transient pulses. After a small interval, called 'recovery time,' the amplifier slowly comes back to the normal condition.

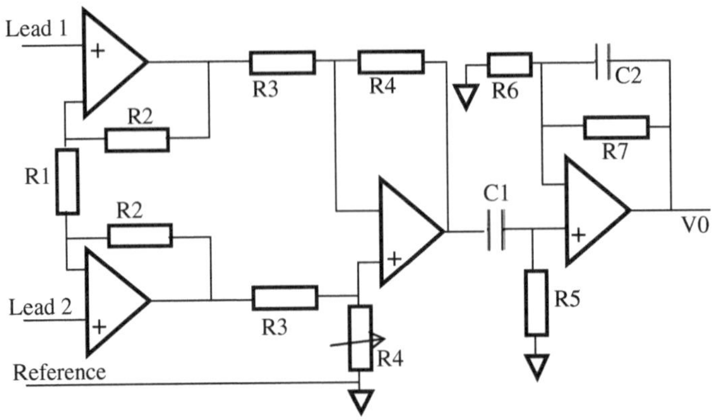

Fig. 3.2 Instrumentation amplifier configuration

5. **Input impedance**: This should be sufficiently high so as to ensure that input signal is not attenuated. Most common ECG amplifiers offer an input impedance of 10 MΩ.
6. **Electrode polarization**: Different varieties of Ag–AgCl electrodes are used for ECG acquisition. The small potential, generated at the electrode–electrolyte interface, is known as half-cell potential. This small DC potential must be considered since it can saturate the INA output, suppressing low-level ECG signal itself. Association for the Advancement of Medical Instrumentation (AAMI) specifies that ECG amplifiers must tolerate a DC component of up to 300 mV resulting in electrode–skin contact.

The popular three-OPAMP configuration is shown in Fig. 3.2 [13], which offers a high CMRR by matched pair of resistors R_3 and R_4. The input stage offers a gain of $(1 + 2R_2/R_1)$, followed by a differential amplifier with gain (R_4/R_3). There is a final stage, which offers a gain of $(1 + R_7/R_6)$.

The third stage uses a filter with bandwidth

$$\Delta f = \frac{1}{2\pi R_7 C_2} - \frac{1}{2\pi R_5 C_1} \tag{3.3}$$

Some more configurations of biopotential amplifier are available in [9]. An important issue is power consumption of INA block. Some monolithic and low-power designs include current balancing and transconductance stage amplifiers, described in [14–17].

In addition to the certain desirable characteristics, specific design enhancements are required, depending on the concerned biosignal:

1. **Electrical interference reduction**: This is mainly contributed by PLI, RF from transmitters, and electrical appliances. Stray capacitances are formed between the ECG lead wires and power lines. The displacement currents flow to ground

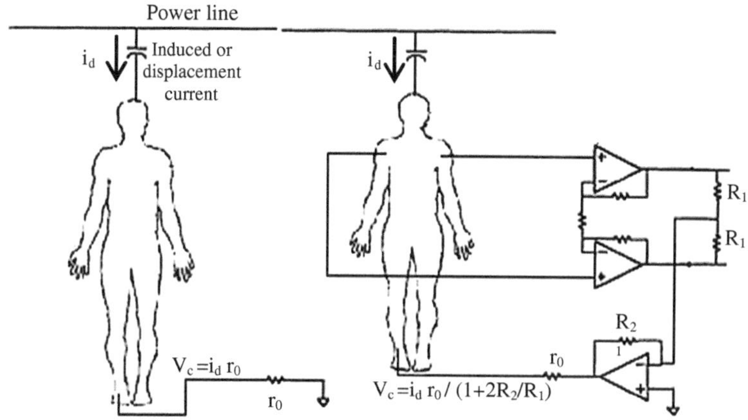

Fig. 3.3 Effect of PLI in ECG measurements and DRL circuit

through the patient body and right leg, which is used as reference. Considering a small resistance r_0 of common lead wire (at right leg) and displacement current i_d, the small drop $V_c = r_0 \, i_d$ appears as common to first stage of INA. A high-CMRR INA can minimize this effect. Additionally, a driven leg circuit (DRL) is used [13, 18], as shown in Fig. 3.3.

In DRL circuit, two sensing registers (R_1) are used to invert, amplify, and feedback the voltage V_c to the right leg of the patient. The modified common-mode voltage becomes

$$V_c = \frac{i_d r_0}{1 + 2R_2/R_1} \tag{3.4}$$

Hence, the interference signal is minimized at the amplifier input. An IC for DRL circuit is described in [19].

2. **Patient isolation**: The objective of patient safety is a biosignal measurement application to ensure that current from the acquisition circuit or its applied part can flow through the patient body to ground, termed 'leakage current,' which remains within safe levels in case of a fault. Thus, all biomedical amplifiers must satisfy some safety criteria for the worst-case voltage breakdown and maximum leakage currents through the input leads attached to the human body. The accepted international standard is IEC-601 for Medical Electrical Equipment adopted by Europe as EN-60601. This is combined with to UL (Underwriters Laboratories Inc.) standard 2601-1 for the United States [20] and endorsed by health industry manufacturers association (HEMA) and national electrical manufacturers association (NEMA) and US Food and Drug Administration (FDA). IEC-60601-1 standard allows a patient auxiliary current (current that can flow between two separate leads connected to the patient

body) up to 100 μA at not less than 0.1 Hz. Normally, patient safety is achieved in two ways, viz., providing complete galvanic isolation between the patient and acquisition circuit (or biomedical equipment) and using surge protection arising from defibrillator or electrosurgical equipment [21]. Galvanic isolation is achieved by electrically separating the input stage of the isolation amplifier (IsoA) from the output stage. That is, the input stage has a separate floating power supply and a 'ground' that are connected to the output side of the IsoA by a high resistance (around 1,000 MΩ) and a low parallel capacitance (around picofarad range). The signal terminals of the input stage are isolated from the IsoA's output by similar high impedance. An IsoA is realized by any of the following techniques, viz. (1) isolation transformer through high-frequency magnetic coupling, (2) optical isolation using LED–phototransistor combination, and (3) capacitive coupling using a signal modulated high-frequency digital carrier from the input stage (isolated) through a pair of capacitors to a demodulator at the output stage.

In transformer isolation, transformer with a toroidal core is used to couple high-frequency (around 500 kHz) AC power from output to isolated input stages where it is rectified and filtered. The output from the isolated phase modulates an AC carrier magnetically coupled to a demodulator at the output stage [22]. Using magnetic isolation, a breakdown voltage of 7 kV can be achieved. Optical isolation uses either linear analog photo-optic coupling or digital modulation of the amplified signal. However, in optical coupling, separate isolated power supply is required to the input stages through high-frequency isolation amplifiers. Linear analog photo-optic coupling can be implemented one infrared LED, optically coupled with two identical phototransistors, either photoconductive or photovoltaic mode of operation. Figure 3.4 shows schematic circuit of LOC 110 linear optocouplers from Clare Inc. [23], operated in photoconductive mode. One phototransistor (T_1) provides a servo feedback to stabilize the LED (D) driving circuit current, and the other (T_2) one provides the galvanic isolation between input and output. The basic operation of the circuit is given as follows:

As the input V_{IN} increases, I_F increases and D starts to conduct. The incident optical flux on T_1 causes a current I_1 to flow, which in turn increases the voltage at inverting terminal of OPAMP U1 by a drop I_1R_1. The voltage V_A at non-inverting terminal gradually becomes equal to V_{IN}, and then, no further increase in I_F occurs. Thus, for a particular I_F, the circuit generated a fixed current I_2 (the output of T_2), which is proportional to LED flux and hence equal to I_1. Hence, the output of the amplifier is given as

$$V_{\text{OUT}} = I_2R_2 = \frac{V_{\text{IN}}}{R_1}R_2 \tag{3.5}$$

Using optical coupling, a breakdown voltage up to 4–7 kV can be achieved. In capacitive IsoA, an internal oscillator is used to modulate the analog differential signal to a digital pulse train, which is transmitted across the isolation barrier, built around a matched pair of capacitors (1–3 pfd range). At the output stage, the

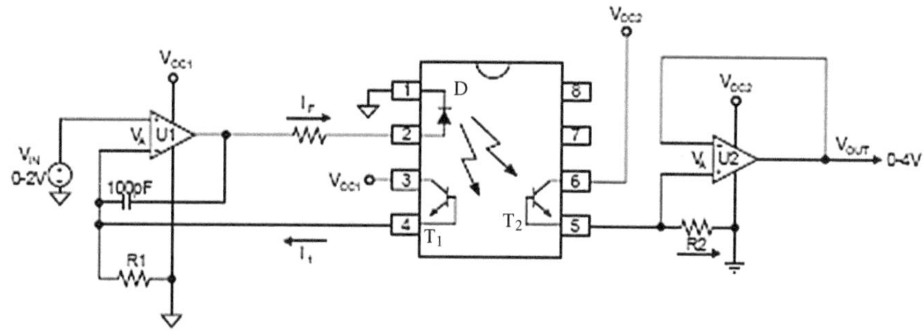

Fig. 3.4 Optical isolation circuit using LOC 110

modulated signal is converted back to analog voltage by an averaging technique. The functional block diagram of a capacitive IsoA is shown in Fig. 3.5. However, in capacitive isolation also, the use of separate isolated power supply is mandatory. In some variants of capacitive IsoA, the input is modulated to a duty cycle encoded signal (Burr-Brown ISO103, ISO107, ISO121), while in others, it is converted to frequency (Burr-Brown ISO102, ISO106).

The performance of an isolation amplifier is described by isolation-mode rejection ratio (IMRR), which refers to its ability to suppress the feed-through isolation-mode voltage that arises across the barrier and output stage, detailed in [24].

Accidental voltage surge protection from the biomedical equipment can be achieved by connecting voltage-limiting devices (e.g., zener diode) between the connecting electrode and ground. The device absorbs the extra current inrush when the voltage across it raises a certain value, typically 300 mV or higher.

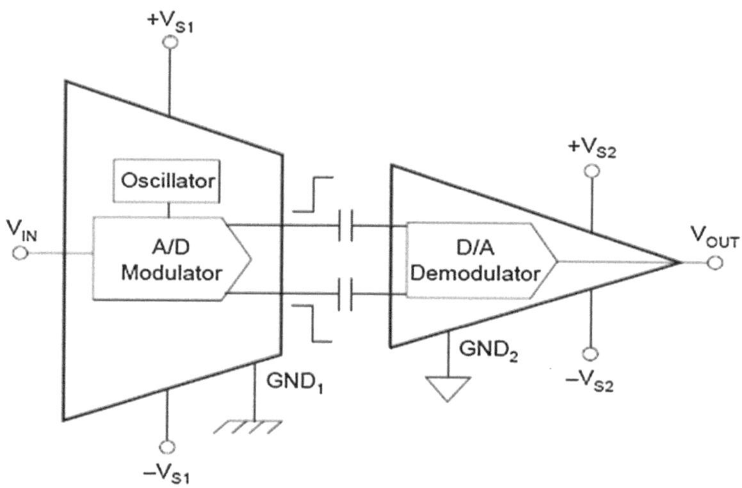

Fig. 3.5 Block diagram of capacitive isolation amplifier

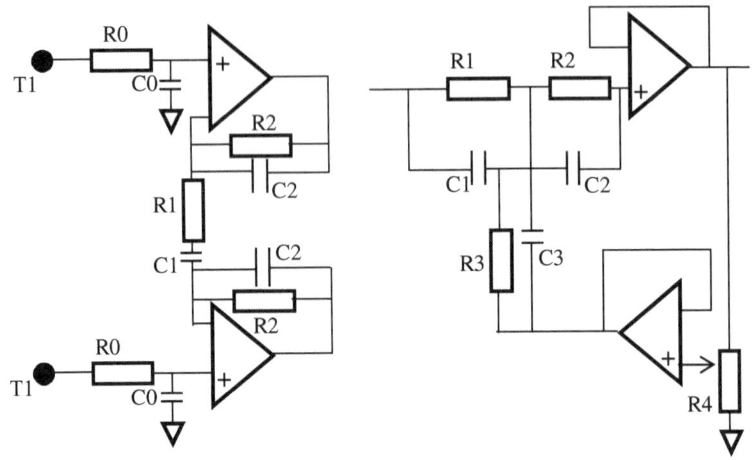

Fig. 3.6 Filtering for noise reduction. **a** Band-pass filtering. **b** Twin-T notch filter for 50-Hz noise reduction

3. **Filtering**: Filtering at the first stage of the amplifier can greatly reduce the unwanted interference. This is shown in Fig. 3.6. Small inductors and ferrite beads (indicated as *T*1) in the lead wires help to block high-frequency electromagnetic interference. *C*0 and *R*0 connected at the lead wire reduce radio frequency interference [13].

Additionally, the *C*1 and *R*1 constitute a high-pass filter and *C*2 and *R*2 the low-pass filter, with an effective bandpass given as

$$fc = \frac{1}{2\pi}\left(\frac{1}{R_1C_1} - \frac{1}{R_2C_2}\right) \tag{3.6}$$

For power line frequency rejection, an adjustable quality twin-*T* notch filter is used where the tuning frequency is given as

$$f_0 = \frac{1}{2\pi R_1 C_1} \tag{3.7}$$

where $R_1 = R_2 = 2R_3$; $C_1 = C_2 = C_3/2$.

3.4 A Single-Channel ECG Acquisition System

As mentioned in Sect. 3.2, the trend is to use customized DAS cards and application software in ECG acquisition systems in clinical setup. The immediate advantages are as follows: easy data storage and retrieval, data sharing in digital format, and computerized analysis. In this section, a stand-alone DAS card

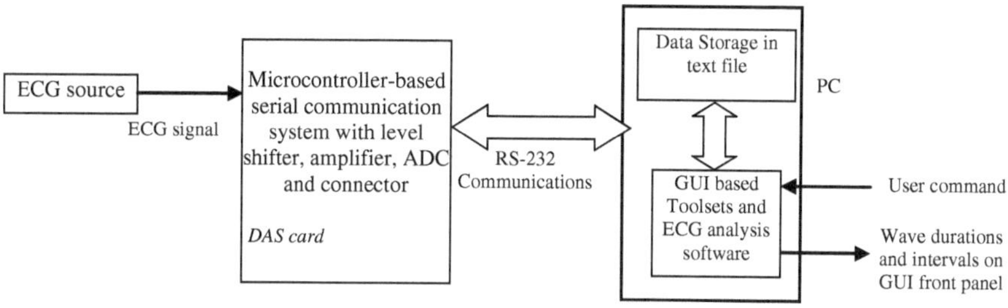

Fig. 3.7 Block diagram of the PC-based ECG DAS

developed by us for single-channel ECG acquisition and computer-based analysis is described. The system is useful for preliminary level diagnosis of a cardiac patient in a health care unit. An 8051 MCU-based stand-alone DAS card is developed, which transmits the ECG samples using the serial port of the PC [25]. A short-duration data (6–8 beats) are acquired for offline analysis using application software, which is developed in MATLAB platform. A graphical user interface provides soft switches and menu-driven front end for easy operation to the user. The functional block diagram of the developed system is shown in Fig. 3.7.

The DAS card contains an analog front end, single-channel AD converter, and an AT89C51 MCU to convert the ECG samples into a serial data stream conforming RS-232 protocol. The serial data stream is transmitted at a speed of 19.2 kbps to the PC for temporary storage in a data file (*.txt format). Finally, a time-stamped data file is generated for time-plane analysis of samples for feature extraction. The extracted time-plane features along with a lead data plot are generated on the GUI front panel.

3.5 Serial Communication Between DAS Card and Computer

3.5.1 Basics of Serial Communication

Over the years, serial port has become the popular choice for communication between embedded systems or between embedded systems and PC. Most of the laboratory-based DAS employs one or other form of serial communication protocol for transmission of sensor's signal to the host PC. The most important features of serial communications are as follows:

1. Saves cable cost, since only two/three wires are enough to achieve full-duplex communication.

2. Data can be transmitted over long distance (e.g., 4,000 feel using RS-485 communication) with a good speed (e.g., 3.2 Gbps using IEEE-1394b or FireWire).

Many of the DAQ hardware manufacturers use a serial communication interface layer between the DAS card and the PC. This communication interface may be one of the protocols like RS-232, RS-485, RS-422, Ethernet, PCI, I2C, 1-wire.

The RS-232 standard, recommended by Electronics Industries Association (EIA) in 1961, is one of the simple and popular serial communication protocols used. The terminology reflects the RS-232 as a standard for communication between a computer terminal and an external device (CRO, modem, etc.) separated by a distance limit of 130 feet. Currently published by Telecommunications Industry Association (TIA), it defines the two devices connected with a serial cable as the data terminal equipment (DTE) and data communication equipment (DCE). The RS-232 standard defines the parameters, viz. electrical characteristic (i.e., signal levels), pin assignments, names and functions of signals, and mechanical specifications. The original specifications use 25 lines of the communication channel; however, most of the real-world devices use a reduced 9-line version, as detailed in Table 3.1.

The connection schematic for RS-232 standard is shown in Fig. 3.8, where the two devices are connected by a serial cable. To implement asynchronous serial transfer, primary communication is accomplished using three pins, viz. the transmit data pin, the receive data pin, and the ground pin. The commonly used version of RS-232 connector is shown in Fig. 3.9, called 'D' connectors.

Using the asynchronous protocol, each communication device uses its own internal clock, resulting in bytes that are transferred at arbitrary times. So, instead of using time as a way to synchronize the bits, a data format (called 'frame') is used. A generalized data format for RS-232 protocol includes a 'low' start bit, 8 data bits, a 'high' stop bit, and a parity bit (optional) as shown in Fig. 3.10.

In RS-232 standard, all signals are specified between the communicating devices, viz. DTE, which receives the data and DCE that initiates communication. However, the signal names are referenced to DTE. For example, TD is an output to

Table 3.1 Serial port pin and signal assignments

Pin	Label	Signal name	Signal type
1	CD	Carrier detect	Control
2	RD	Receive data	Data
3	TD	Transmit data	Data
4	DTR	Data terminal ready	Control
5	GND	Signal ground	Control
6	DSR	Dataset ready	Control
7	RTS	Request to send	Control
8	CTS	Clear to send	Control
9	RI	Ring indicator	Control

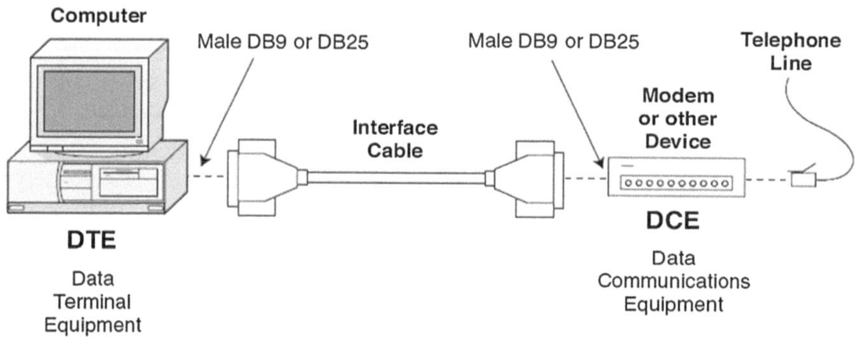

Fig. 3.8 Block diagram of the RS-232 connection system

Fig. 3.9 9 pin RS-232 sockets

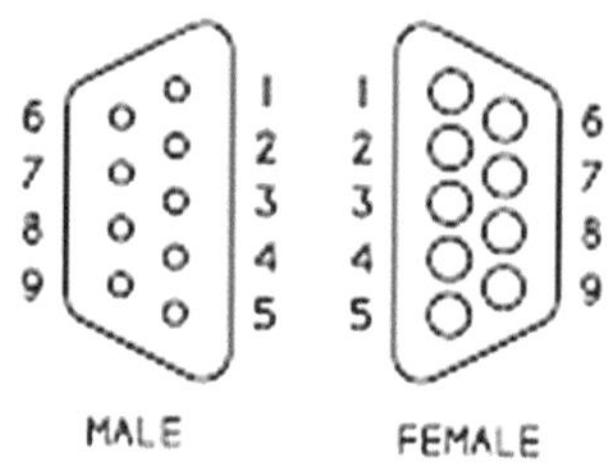

DTE and input to DCE. In most of the transfer operations, DTE is a personal computer and DCE may be either modem, embedded system, or another computer.

RS-232 standard used positive and negative voltage levels, rather than positive voltage levels described by TTL or CMOS logic. Logic '1' (or high) is represented by −12 V, while logic '0' (or low) by +12 V. These levels are chosen to avoid the noise levels and attenuation of signals at the end of a long communication link. At the receiver, a voltage greater than +3 V is regarded as a logic '0' (low) and −3 V as logic '1' (high), an undefined between these two.

For communication between RS-232 and real-world devices (which operate on TTL logic or CMOS logic), a level converter IC is used in the transceiver circuits. Most common ICs are MAX232 and MAX233 from Maxim Corporation. Further details of serial communications can be obtained in [26].

3.5.2 *Serial Communication Using 8051 Microcontroller-Based DAS Card*

The detail schematic of the hardware test setup for developed ECG acquisition system is given in Fig. 3.11. The ECG signal is generated by an arbitrary waveform generator (AWG) and model Agilent A33220A in conjunction with Agilent Intuilink Waveform editor, fed with PhysioNet data [27].

	D0	D1	D2	…	…	…	…	D7			
Start bit	Data bits								Parity bit	Stop bits	

Fig. 3.10 Data frame format in RS-232 protocol

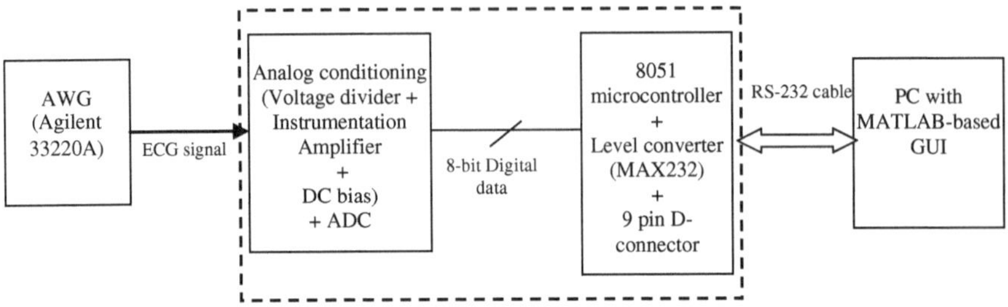

Fig. 3.11 Detailed schematic of the DAQ hardware

Agilent Intuilink Waveform editor provides a software platform to generate any kind of voltage waveform when the data samples of a complete period are provided in a normalized scale. The peak amplitude and frequency of the generated waveform can be set from the menu panels. If the data samples with amplitude and time period setting are downloaded to the volatile memory of the AWG, it generates (and repeats) the analog signal continuously. To generate different types of normal and abnormal ECG signals, precise R–R interval data from respective lead are used as described.

The single-channel ADC0804 is used in continuous conversion mode and sampled at 1 kHz by the MCU to comply with the frequency of ptb-db database. Each sampled data are converted to RS-232-formatted data and delivered at a speed of 19.2 kbps to the PC for serial acquisition in a text file. So, considering a 10-bit frame (one start bit, 8 data bits, and 1 stop bit), each transfer consumes 520 μs for complete reception at PC universal serial asynchronous receiver/transmitter (USART). The time frame activity of the serial link is shown in Fig. 3.12. Thus, between two successive ADC sampling, the link remains idle for 480 μs. The Atmel 89C52 MCU is programmed at mode 1 communitarian which is similar to RS-232 protocol. The flowchart for MCU is given in Appendix 1 at the end of this chapter.

3.5.3 Serial Communication in MATLAB Environment

MATLAB supports direct data transfer between two devices TIA/EIA-232 standard published by TIA. A generalized data flow (input) diagram involving the serial port in PC and the DAS card is shown in Fig. 3.13.

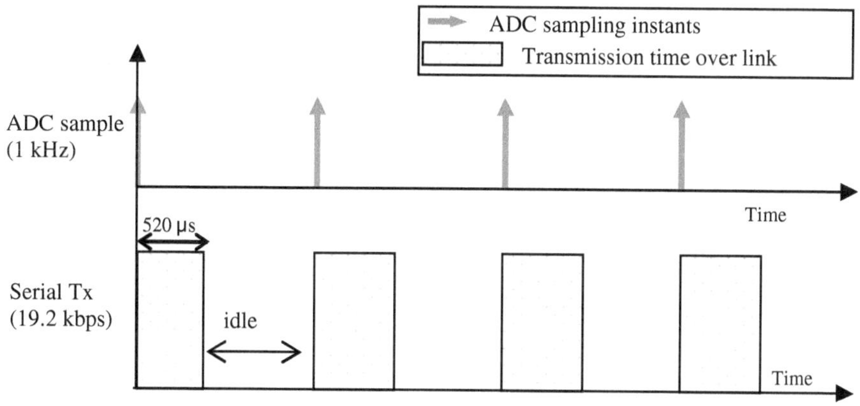

Fig. 3.12 Timescale activity of serial link versus ADC sampling

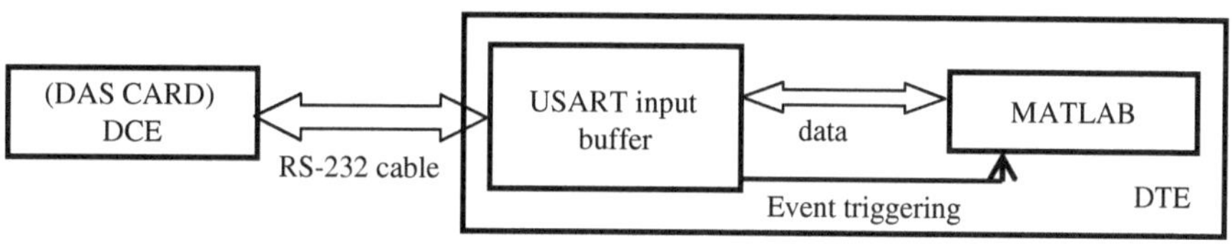

Fig. 3.13 Data flow schematic between MATLAB and DAQ hardware

Most traditional PCs are provided with one or more serial ports (popularly known as 'COM' or communication port), which contain a USART IC as the interface between the application software and the external world. A portion of the computer memory is allocated as input and output buffer associated with the same USART. The memory size allocated to this buffer can be changed through software instructions. As shown in Fig. 3.10, the data exchange between DCE (here stand-alone DAS card) and the PC takes place through the same buffer. It serially transfers out the data from the output buffer memory to the external device or receive data from external device through input buffer with the specified baud rate.

For data transfer operations with the external work using the serial port, a tool is provided to access the USART through a 'serial' object, which can be directly created in MATLAB platform to achieve real-time communication. All properties of this 'serial' object can be changed using MATLAB commands. For seamless transfer of data with external DAS card, the principle of 'event-driven programming' is used, which provides a programmer to access the USART buffer for data input/output based on certain 'event' generated in real-time operation using MATLAB commands.

For a typical data input process, the following sequence of events take place:

1. Data from the external device (stand-alone DAS card) continuously fill up the input buffer of the USART using the RD line;

2. When input buffer filling reaches predefined (user programmable) threshold value, then it generates an 'event,' which triggers the corresponding MATLAB callback functions using 'bytes-available event';
3. Data are picked up from buffer using necessary command in MATLAB.

For transferring data bytes to the outside world, an exact reverse sequence is executed, as stated below:

1. From computer memory, data byes are sent to the output buffer of the USART using commands in MATLAB;
2. The USART continuously transmits the data bytes to the external device using the TD line;
3. An 'OutputEmpty' event is generated when the output buffer goes empty, triggering the corresponding event described by 'BytesAvailableFcn' and 'OutputEmptyFcn.' The calling function loads the next block of data to the USART for delivery to the external device.

A typical session for using serial port objects involves the following steps to be initiated using software instructions:

1. Creating a serial port object using 'serial' creation function.
2. Opening the port.
3. Setting the following properties related to the serial port functions:
   - Baud rate
   - Parity
   - Data bits
   - Stop bits
   - Input buffer size
   - 'ReadAsyncMode' which describes manual/automatic mode for reading the port for data availability
   - 'BytesAvailableFcn' describes the function which will be called every time an event described by 'BytesAvailableFcnMode' property is generated
   - 'BytesAvailableFcnCount' describes the number of bytes which when available in the input buffer will generate the callback event.
4. Picking up (or deliver) the data bytes available in the buffer in (or from) a data array.
5. Closing the port.

The incoming data to the PC serial port are sequentially stored in a text file. These data are in the range 0–255, i.e., 8-bit quantization. To enable data storage in actual ECG sample, a conversion formula is used as

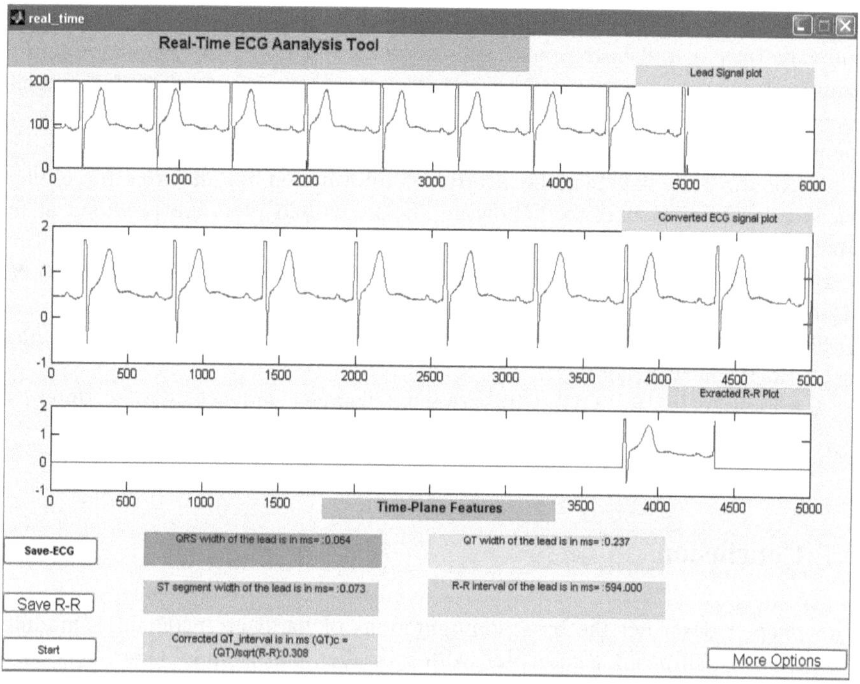

Fig. 3.14 Developed GUI for PC-based ECG acquisition

$$\text{Analog(mV) value } (V_a) = \frac{[\text{Digital value (D)} - \text{digital equivalent of bias voltage}] \times 19.6}{\text{Total amplification achieved in Amplifiers}} \tag{3.8}$$

where 19.6 mV corresponds to the resolution of the ADC.

The flowchart of the MATLAB algorithm is given in Appendix 2. The lead data are finally stored in a two-column time-stamped data file for future processing.

3.6 GUI-Based Front End for ECG Acquisition System

Nowadays, graphical user interfaces have become an integral part of any application software. MATLAB provides an easy-to-develop platform with most common tools for graphical user interface development. Hence, a user interface developed in MATLAB provides additional advantage of using the powerful computational tools. In recent years, there has been extensive use of MATLAB GUI in biomedical applications [28–29]. In the developed ECG DAS as described in Sects. 3.4, 3.5, the objective is to provide a simple easy to interface to the operator at the healthcare clinic for collection of patients' ECG. The interface contains some MATLAB-based soft keys, menus, and toolsets. The application software runs in the background and has dual functions: first, collecting ECG samples from the stand-alone DAS and storing it in a time-stamped data file and second, extracting time-plane features from a collected lead data and displaying them in a meaningful manner on the GUI for easy interpretation. Added with this, a plot of the lead data will be additional information for the user for clinical decision making. Hence, the following signatures and plots are provided at the front panel:

ECG time-plane features are as follows: 1. R–R interval; 2. QRS interval; 3. ST segment width; 4. QT interval; and 5. corrected Qt interval or $(QT)_c$.

Plots are as follows: 1. lead plot of quantized data; 2. reconstructed data plot; and 3. R–R interval plot.

A screenshot of the GUI with extracted features and lead plot is shown in Fig. 3.14.

3.7 Conclusion

This chapter describes the basic configurations of hardware acquisition modules for ECG acquisitions in a computer, with special emphasis on ECG artifacts, ECG amplifiers, and their design requirements, followed by an ECG acquisition system with the development of a stand-alone embedded system used as DAS card. A brief introduction on serial communication protocols, signal characteristics, and its implementation between the DAS card and MATLAB-based application software is provided.

Acknowledgments Paper [25] is the contribution from Biomedical Signal acquisition and Processing Research Group at Department of Applied Physics, University of Calcutta, India.

End of Chapter Appendix 1

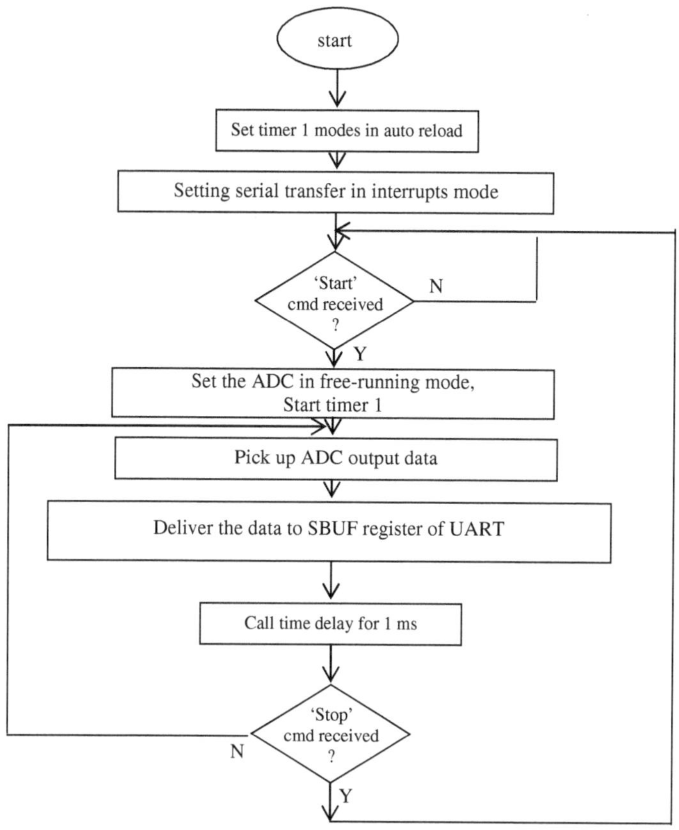

End of Chapter Appendix 2

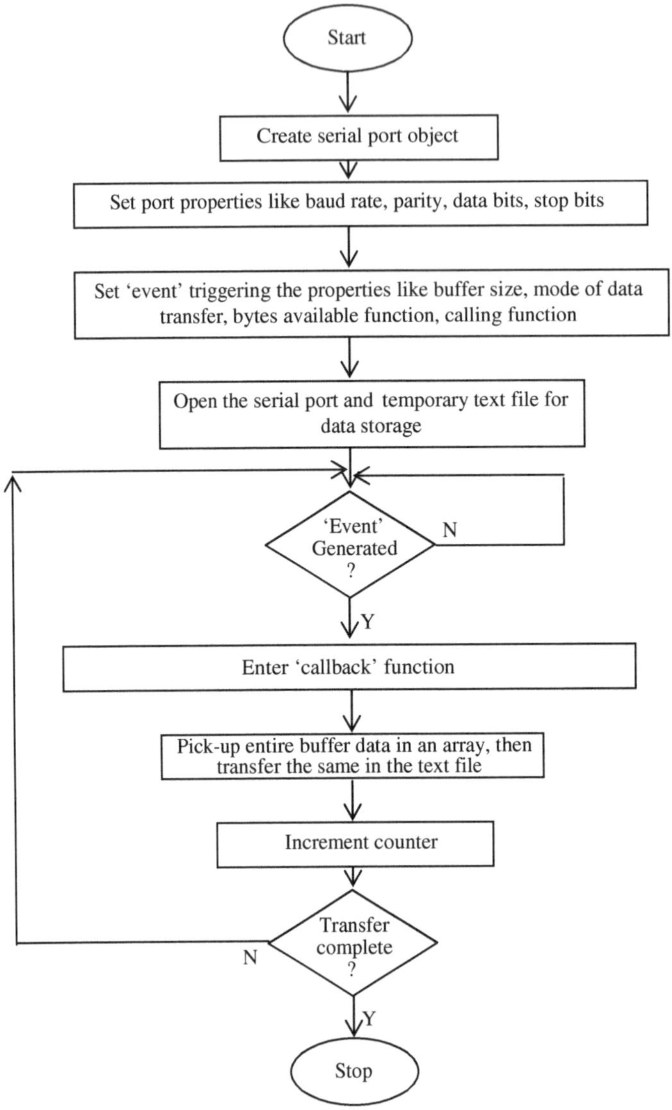

References

1. Plonsey R, Barr RC. Bioelectricity: a quantitative approach. 3rd ed. NY, USA: Springer; 2007.
2. Schamroth L. An introduction to electrocardiography. 7th ed. Cambridge: Blackwell Science; 2008.
3. Hampton JR. ECG made easy. 7th ed. UK: Churchill Livingstone; 2008.
4. Huhta JH, Webster JG. 60 Hz interference in electrocardiography. IEEE Trans Biomed Eng. 1973;BME-20(2):91–101.
5. Spinelli EM, Mayosky MA, Areny RP. A practical approach to electrode-skin impedance unbalance measurement. IEEE Trans Biomed Eng. 2006;53(7):1451–3.
6. Ider YZ, Saki MC, Giiger HA. Removal of power line interference in signal-averaged electrocardiography systems. IEEE Trans Biomed Eng. 1995;40(7):731–5.
7. Friesen GM, Jannett TC, Jadallah MA, Yates SL, Quint SR, Nagle HT. A comparison of noise sensitivity of nine QRS detection algorithm. IEEE Trans Biomed Eng. 1990;37(1):85–98.
8. Chaudhury S, Pawar TD, Duttagupta S. Ambulation analysis in wearable ECG. New York: Springer; 2009.
9. Prutchi D, Norris M. Design and development of medical electronic instrumentation: a practical perspective of the design, construction, and test of medical devices. New Jersey: Wiley Interscience; 2005.
10. Areny RP, Webster JG. AC instrumentation amplifier for bioimpedance measurements. IEEE Trans Biomed Eng. 1993;40(8):830–3.
11. Spinelli EM, Areny RP, Myosky MA. AC coupled front end for biopotential measurements. IEEE Trans Biomed Eng. 2003;50(3):391–5.
12. Spinelli EM, Martinez N, Myosky MA, Areny RP. A novel fully differential biopotential amplifier With DC suppression. IEEE Trans Biomed Eng. 2004;51(8):1444–8.
13. Webster JG, ed. Measurement, sensors and instrumentation handbook. New York: CRC press LLC.
14. Steyaert M, Sansen W. A micropower low-noise monolithic instrumentation amplifier for medical purposes. IEEE J Solid-State Circuits. 1987;22(6):1163–8.
15. Krabbe H. A high-performance monolithic instrumentation amplifier. IEEE international conference in solid-state circuits XIV, 17–19 Feb 1971. Pennsylvania, pp. 186–187.
16. Martins R, Selberherr S, Vaz F. A CMOS IC for portable EEG acquisition systems. IEEE Trans Instrum Meas. 1998;47(5):1191–6.
17. Brokaw A, Timko M. An improved monolithic instrumentation amplifier. IEEE J Solid-State Circuits. 1975;10(6):417–23.
18. Webster JG, ed. Medical instrumentation: application and design. 4th ed. New York: Wiley; 2010.
19. Wong A, Pun KP, Zhang YP, Choy CS. An ECG measurement IC circuit using driven right leg circuit. IEEE international symposium on circuits and systems 2006, 21–24 May 2006. Greece, pp. 345–348.
20. Medical electrical equipment–part 1: general requirements for basic safety and essential performance from international electrotechnical commission website.
21. Bronzino JD, ed. The biomedical engineering handbook. 2nd ed. New York: CRC Press LLC.
22. Data sheet of transformer-coupled hybrid isolation amplifier model 3656.
23. Clare Inc liner Optocouplers 110 data sheet.
24. van Rijn ACM, Peper A, Grimbergen CA. The isolation mode rejection ratio in bioelectric amplifiers'. IEEE Trans Biomed Eng. 1991;38(11):1154–7.
25. Gupta R, Bera JN, Mitra M. Development of an embedded system and MATLAB-based GUI for online acquisition and analysis of ECG signal. Measurement (Elsevier). 2010;43(9):1119–26.

26. Axelson J. Serial port complete: COM Ports, USB virtual COM ports, and ports for embedded systems. 2nd ed. Madison, WI: Lakeview Research LLC.
27. PhysioNet database. http://www.physionet.org/.
28. Schwarzenberg GF, Zapf M, Ruiter NV. A MATLAB GUI for the analysis and exploration of signal and image of an ultrasound computer tomograph, in: first international conference on advances in computer-human interaction (ACHI-2008), 10–15 Feb 2008. Sent Luce, Martinique, pp. 53–58.
29. Chaibi S, Bouet R, Jung J, Lajnef T, Samet L, Bertrand O, KAchouri A, Jerbi K. Development of matlab-based graphical user interface (GUI) for detection of high frequency oscillations (HFOs) in epileptic patients. IEEE international conference on emerging signal processing applications (ESPA), 12–14 Jan 2012. Las Vegas, USA, pp. 56–62.

Chapter 4
ECG Transmission

4.1 Introduction

The last few decades witnessed tremendous developments in Information and Communication Technologies (ICT), mainly in the area of public networks, speed of access, data security, and accessibility of channels. A major application of ICT is evidenced in tele-healthcare, which deals with transmission of medical data from the subject to a remote place for storage and analysis. Tele-cardiology, a special branch of telemedicine, involves transmission of patient's cardiac information (ECG, echo images, catheter images etc.,) for remote-end acquisition, analysis, interpretation by experts and feedback. The increasing quality and fidelity of transmitted biomedical data added with user-friendly interfaces have provided the opportunity of real-life experience of physical consultation with medical experts. With the advent of VLSI technology, backed by high-end, low-power processors, biomedical signals are now possible to be acquired in handheld devices (like mobile phones, PDA etc.,) and often, transmitted to healthcare centre or medical professional directly for expert advice and further actions through various public networks. Thus, the healthcare service, empowered by various data communication techniques is no more confined to healthcare clinics or hospitals. This chapter provides a brief review of different ECG transmission techniques. Finally, a prototype system developed as a low-cost alternative for providing tele-cardiology service is described.

4.2 Review of ECG Transmission Techniques

Historically, the first instance of communication in healthcare took place at the end of eighteenth century, when Willem Einthoven carried out experimentations on patients' ECG transmission from the nearby hospital to his laboratory using post office telephone lines. Although the technological developments have taken place in manifolds since the Einthoven's era, the general principles of tele-ECG have

R. Gupta et al., *ECG Acquisition and Automated Remote Processing*,
DOI: 10.1007/978-81-322-1557-8_4, © Springer India 2014

remained the same. Following his study, there were many applications of patients' physiological data transmission, mainly over public switched telephone network (PSTN) lines. The earlier tele-cardiology systems used analog signal processing systems and frequency modulation (FM) for single-channel ECG acquisition or frequency division multiplexing (FDM) system for multilead acquisition [1]. With the introduction of computer programs for ECG interpretation, most of these applications were centered on transferring of patients' ECG data from hospitals to computer laboratories. In [2] a comparison between analog FDM transmission and digital time, division multiplexing (TDM) is described in the context of technical (such as real time or offline transmission, bandwidth, accuracy etc.) and economic (like overall cost) considerations for a transmission length of 20 miles. For analog transmission, three centre frequencies of 1.075, 1.935, and 2.365 kHz were used. The functional block diagram of such analog transmission system is shown in Fig. 4.1. Analog transmission approaches suffered from corruption of the signal due to poor quality of the transmission lines, low immunity to line impulse noise, inadequate processing and incompatibility with computer communication protocols at the receiving end. This raised a question of the reliability of the signal for clinical use, specially for computer-assisted diagnosis. In addition, limitation of the then PSTN bandwidth (300–3,400 Hz) was also a hindrance toward transmission of low-frequency ECG signal. Initially, the major problem with digital transmission was found to be with low data rate (around 9,600 bps in UK) for 3-lead multiplexed ECG transmission. However, with the development of high-end communication gadgets, these problems were gradually overcome later on.

With the introduction of digital technology, viz., easy computer interfacing without demodulation, multiplexing and AD conversion and improved signal quality due to error detection capability, communication gadgets (like synchronous modems) were used at the transmitting end for digital ECG transmission. However, to accommodate 3-lead multiplexed ECG over switched network using low-cost modems for a sampling rate of 200 sps, the acquired ECG data had either to be compressed (or encoded) or transmitted offline. An application of numerical ECG encoding by delta encoding using Intellec-8 MOD08 microcomputer is described [3]. The method used a low-cost modem using 2,400 bps coupled with a telephone network. Although digital transmission crept in additional characters as control frames, the overall accuracy and performed obtained were better than analog FM transmission. From the advent of wireless communication techniques in 1970s, there was a gradual shift in choice of transmission media. The first instance of mobile tele-cardiology was reported in 1970, which provided remote means of acquisition and transmission of patients' ECG using conventional radio equipment. Added with this, advent of VLSI technology enabled use of high-speed processors for complex digital processing of data. A major application of the microcomputer-based systems was evidenced in medical equipments, communication systems, and personal computer (PC) technology [4].

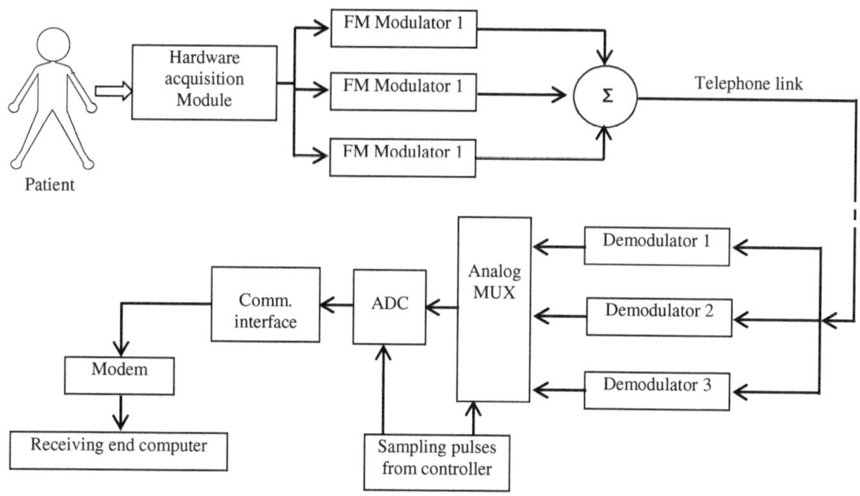

Fig. 4.1 Block schematic of an analog ECG communication system

Tele-ECG applications can be broadly classified based on certain factors, viz., distance of transmission, mobility of the patient and doctor, continuous or intermittent monitoring etc. For short-range communication like patient monitoring in hospitals, embedded systems and low-range radio transmitters are used for real-time ECG transmission. A typical tele-ECG setup consists of three basic functional modules, viz., patient data collector, communication interface, and communicating device at the transmit end. A similar structure with corresponding complement functional blocks at the receiving end completes a computerized acquisition. The patient ECG is collected through a hardware acquisition module (HAM), which consists of lead connectors, ECG amplifiers, filters, isolation circuits followed by a DSP-based microcontroller unit (MCU). Its function is to condition the low-amplitude ECG signal, digitize it and then supply the samples to the communicating device using a suitable protocol. The communicating device may be a mobile phone, PDA, or computer. It applies a data compression algorithm, encodes the compressed data, and finally transmits. Sometimes, the MCU of the HAM performs the compression and source encoding function and directly feeds the data stream to the transmitter module. Works on such prototype system using portable stand-alone embedded systems and low-power commercial FM transmitters are available in the literature. Like, in [5–7], the authors report an 8051 MCU using with FM/FSK transmitter for ECG transmission. In similar applications [8], NI DAQ cards are used for direct acquisition of received data in a laptop or PC along with some processing [9] capability.

Real-time monitoring of cardiac patient applications are divided into two major areas, viz., ambulatory monitoring for chronic patients and home telecare systems. For emergency medical service, ECG transmission of the patients from ambulances was practiced from early 1970s. In [10], a low-cost mobile unit installed in an ambulance is described, which uses communication equipment for simultaneous voice and ECG transmission between the emergency vehicle and nearby hospital. Accordingly, prehospital emergency arrangements could be achieved, and hence, some critical patients with arrhythmia could be saved. A similar study is carried out in [11] for acute myocardial infarction (MI) patients. An offline compression technique of 12-lead ECG is reported in [12], where a portable ECG machine was used for acquiring the ECG data and transmitting through a cellular phone.

Mobile tele-cardiology was also successfully implemented using satellite communication in airborne aircraft and mid-ocean ships to handle an emergency situation arising due to sudden cardiac pain of a passenger. In [13], the authors report functional description and successful implementation of a mobile satellite communication (MSC) for telemedicine services with 3-lead ECG signal and some other vital signs being transmitted along with the voice signals for a real-time consultation with the base station cardiologist, located at a city hospital. The main challenges of MSC are channel capacity (10–100 kbps) to allow multiplexed transmission of data and video signal, data reliability, delay of transmission (which is sometimes 1 s or more) and electromagnetic interference with the navigation system of the moving vehicle itself. With the increasing practice of ECG transmission for various medical services, standard communication protocol (SCP)-ECG was developed in Europe in 1993. The SCP-ECG standard specifies the content and the structure of the information between the transmitting station (mobile cart) and the receiving station (host) for computer-assisted electrocardiography. In [14], an implementation of the protocol for real-time digital transmission of the 12-lead ECG at a speed of 9,600 bps from ambulance car to the nearest hospital is reported. The major challenges faced were time delay (sometimes 2 min) for the initial establishment of the telephone connection and moving/static condition of the vehicle. It was found that the rate of correct reception of the ECG is better when the vehicle is at rest. Similar systems reported [15, 16] were of store and forward type, which means, they cannot be used for real-time monitoring applications. In [17] the authors report a GSM-based real-time system for the transmission of critical biosignals and images from a mobile unit to a dedicated workstation, named 'telemedicine consultation station' acting as the consultation site. The mobile unit collects 12-lead ECG (sampled at 200 sps), SpO_2, heart rate, blood pressure, temperature, images (at 320×240 pixel resolution) and communicated through TCP/IP over GSM at 9.6 kbps. The patient data collected at the workstation are archived at an encrypted database management system for future use. The developed system showed good response with occasional interruption in case of ECG and $Sp0_2$ transmission. The medical expert could advice the paramedic personnel from the consulting site during the patient being transported to hospital.

Another significant development took place in the area of using internet services for remote patient care. This allowed elderly patients to contact the specialists periodically and remote checkup from clinics. In [18], the authors report a web-based system implemented for remote monitoring of vital signs (like ECG, respiration, invasive and non-invasive BP, SpO_2) from a bedside monitor, the IP address of which was obtained from a patient locator service. The patient locator service provided the basic patient information like hospital, ICU/CCU, bed number, etc. This was accessed from the central monitoring server using a message exchange service. The doctor at the server could access any patient's data in real-time environment. An extension of this service is described in [19] where the doctor can instruct the remote attendants near the patients for clinical actions and administer treatments. Here, two different doctors, sitting at different locations can talk with each other in real time with patient's vital signs displayed on their computer screen. Development of a remote diagnosis system using public network is described [20] for monitoring a patient at his daily life. A short-range wireless patient module acquired the ECG and transmitted to a local desktop PC, which again transmitted the same to a remote-end computer using integral services digital network (ISDN) telephone network at a speed of 128 kbps. Along with this, the patient's voice and moving image was transmitted using H.120 video conferencing data compression regulation. A detailed architectural description of web-based ECG monitoring is described in [21]. Another web-based application for remote computerized processing is described in [22]. The system provides a user-friendly interface developed in HTML and MATLAB to access patient's ECG (raw or compressed format) from a remote node (local acquisition PC) and analyze the signal using advanced computational techniques. The analysis results are sent back to the user end PC. MATLAB web server toolbox was used for developing the interface application with the server and MATWEB program was used for communication with MATLAB. A framework for multiple patients monitoring in a web environment using the concept of medical information system (MIS)-ECG is described in [23]. A central database server stored, organized, and managed the patient's ECG picked up from different hospitals using onboard network interface controller (NIC) installed on the hardware acquisition board. This allows a direct TCP/IP conversion of ECG data using a Rabbit microcontroller (RCM2200 core) from the patient module. For patients with significant cardiac abnormalities, an internet-based ECG evaluation and follow-up system is described in [24]. The patient's ECG was compared with prestored validated ECG database containing five major classes and subclasses. The best match was found out with 50 data, and a histogram is constructed with diagnostic probabilities. This provided a suitable quantitative assessment of the unknown ECG. A continuous monitoring system using GSM network for arrhythmia patients is described [25]. The patient's ECG (2-channel) along with pacemaker and SpO_2 were picked up in a mobile phone through an ECG telemetry transmitter (Danica Biomedical make T3300) using RS-232 protocol. The mobile phone transmitted the ECG beats to a remote Teleguard modem server at a speed of 3600 bps. CRC error check and sequence numbers were generated automatically for missed packet estimation. A store and forward type tele-cardiology application in Portugal reports use of standard email services is reported [26].

4.3 Scheme of ECG Transmission

In this section, an ECG transmission technique is illustrated which may be utilized for remote offline monitoring of patients between two fixed stations. The developed system utilizes portable embedded system–based modules, placed at the two end of the transmission link. The transmit-end module collects the ECG samples from the ECG source and communicates them using a suitable modulation technique using an active media for remote-end reception. At the receive end, another embedded system coupled with the receiver unit decodes the samples and delivers them to a desktop computer for storage and analysis using state of the art software. Thus, the entire system constitutes by the following components:

1. Portable tele-cardiology kit (PTK) as the collecting device from the ECG source, encoding, and data packaging with error checking protocol for transmission;
2. Transmitters and receivers;
3. Healthcare End Embedded System (HES) for the decoding of ECG received from receiver unit, modification of packets for bit error rate (BER) and packet error (PE) computation and serial delivery to the PC;
4. PC-based ECG acquisition and processing system for the serial reception of data, error estimation, saving in time-stamped format, and data processing for ECG feature extraction.

4.3.1 Use of Bi-phase Modulation for ECG Encoding

ECG is a low-frequency signal, primarily in the band 0.05–100 Hz. However, the clinical information is mostly confined within the 30 Hz range. Moreover, except the QRS regions of a typical ECG cycle, the signal change in medium (P and T waves) and very low (equipotential segments like PR, ST, and TP). Bi-phase encoding is a digital encoding scheme suitable for the transmission of such low-frequency signal. It utilizes two distinct frequencies (normally one double of the other) to encode the digital output of the input binary bit stream. In a BPM scheme, as shown in the Fig. 4.2, the output bit always toggles its state after a fixed interval of time. This interval of time, in other words, determines the bit width of the output bit. Again, depending on the input data bit status, the output level may toggle once in the middle of the bit-width interval. If the input bit is ‘1’, the output undergoes one state transition at the middle of that interval, while for ‘0’ bit, there is no such transition. This implies that the frequency to represent a ‘1’ bit is exactly double to that of ‘0’ bit. So, in general, a bi-phase modulation is a special type of FSK (Frequency Shift Keying) modulation [27]. For successive occurrence of same bit at input, there will be a state transition between two intervals at the output. By this way, during transmission, dc like nature of the original ADC

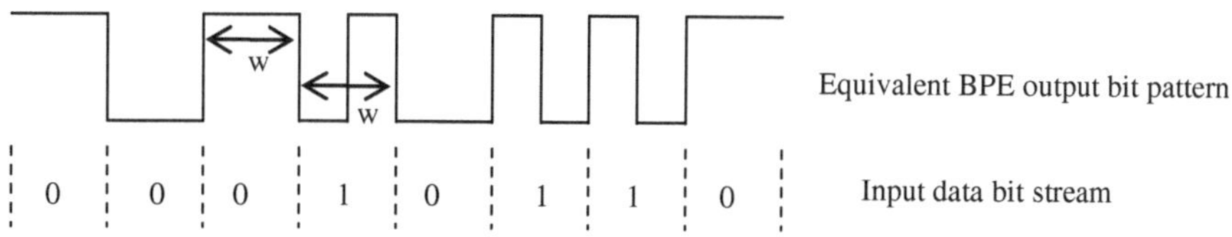

Fig. 4.2 Bi-phase modulation principle illustrated

output, which may occur due to successive '0' or '1' bits, is avoided, instead a continuous time varying signal is generated at the output of the encoder device.

4.3.2 *Standalone Embedded Systems for ECG Encoding and Decoding*

As already mentioned, there are two standalone systems, viz., PTK and HES which are placed at the two ends of the transmission link [28]. The PTK consists of analog signal conditioning modules, a single channel AD converter, Atmel 89C51 MCU, 32 kB SRAM for onboard buffering of ECG samples and driving circuit for transmitter. The analog signal conditioning block consists of a low-offset instrumentation amplifier (INA) followed by a DC shifting arrangement to make the amplified output unipolar and hence compatible with the input of ADC 0804, which is driven at free-running mode. The block schematic of the PTK is shown is Fig. 4.3. The sampling frequency of the AD converter is set as 1 kHz. The PTK collects the ECG samples and continuously fills-up the buffer. After the data are stored, the MCU prepares the data packets and error codes for generating the byte-stream to the transmitter unit. Designing the packet stream is done keeping in view of simplicity, ease in implementation and decoding. Each packet is constituted by a one fixed header, one byte packet number, 32 encoded data bytes, and one error checking code. A fixed header (255_{10}) is used for synchronization between the transceiver units. The packet number is used for BER and PE computation. A typical packet format is shown in Fig. 4.4. For the present case, a simple modular checksum principle is used. The algorithm for generating one encoded packet is given in end of Chapter Appendix 1. Each encoded byte is further formatted with a 'LOW' start bit, 8 data bits and a 'HIGH' stop bit to form the data frame. Precise bit width in the MCU is generated by using two dedicated delay subroutines, each for bit '1' and bit '0'. The output bit line of the MCU is complemented at the end of respective delays which are executed as per the bit's status of a particular frame.

HES receives the demodulated output from the receiver unit and decodes then real time to extract the data frames, then transfers the data bytes to the standalone computer using RS-232 protocol. The block schematic of HES unit is shown in Fig. 4.5 [29]. The output of the receiver is in sinusoidal form, and hence, a wave shaping circuit is used for converting it into an equivalent binary bit stream which

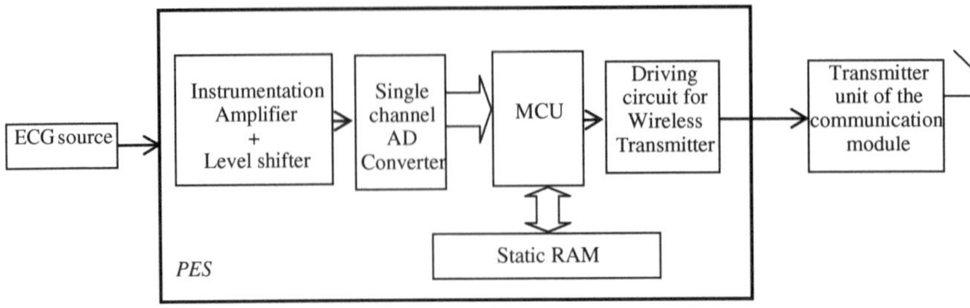

Fig. 4.3 Block schematic of the PTK

Header	Packet number	Encoded data bytes (1-32)	Checksum byte
'sync pattern'			

Fig. 4.4 Structure of a transmitted 35-byte packet from PES

is delivered to the MCU (Atmel 89C2051). The decoding of input data stream is performed by accurate computation of the bit intervals between successive state transitions using the timer elements of the MCU. The timer element compares this bit interval value with a reference level and the decoded bit status is assigned. A '0' bit is encoded from one wider pulse and '1' bit from two consecutive thinner pulses. The algorithm flowchart of this decoding is given in end of Chapter Appendix 2.

Initially, the HES MCU looks for a match of the 'header' pattern from the decoded frames, and when it is found, it accepts the subsequent bytes for further processing. For each decoded frame, the start and stop bits are selectively discarded to extract the data byte only in the following manner. From the point of matching, the last 8 bits out of 10 (a complete frame) are accepted for all successive decoded data frames. This automatically discards the stop bit of preceding frame and start bit of the following frame, as indicated in Fig. 4.6. The next function is to modify the decoded packets for BER and PE estimation. For this, a

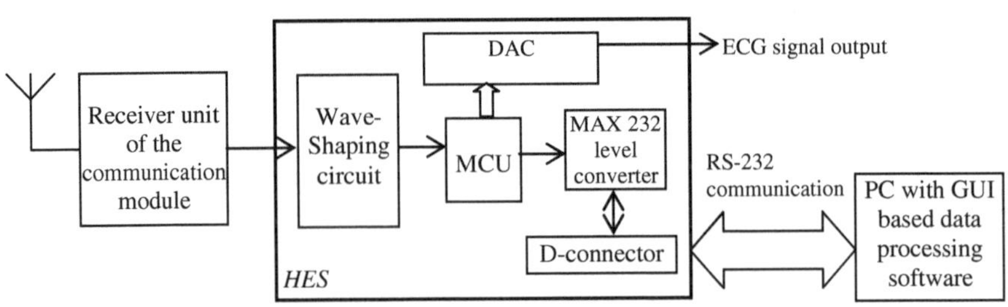

Fig. 4.5 Block schematic of the HES module

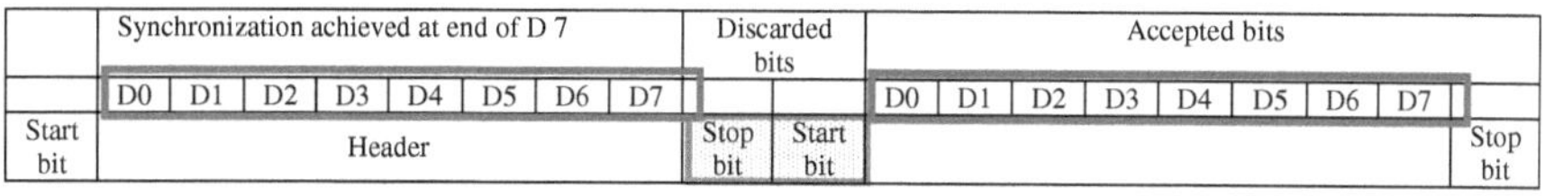

Fig. 4.6 Principle of byte recovery from decoded frame

'checksum error' byte is generated by the MCU from each decoded packet of the received data by sequentially adding all the 35 bytes (header, packet number, data bytes, and checksum byte). For an error free communication, this 'checksum error' byte should be zero for each received packet. The checksum byte (i.e., the last byte) of each received packet is replaced by the corresponding 'checksum error' byte while being delivered to the PC, keeping other bytes intact. So, each received packet is custom-made to form a 'modified packet'. In the PC, an estimation of communication error can be performed by checking the last byte (which is 'checksum error' byte) of each packet. The algorithms steps for generating the checksum error byte from received packets from the point of achieving synchronization in the HES MCU is given in end of Chapter Appendix 3.

The HES firmware incorporates an intelligence to recover from an occasional link failure between the transceiver units. In such situations, the input line of HES MCU becomes temporarily 'locked', without any transition, at a level (high or low) for certain period which is much greater than LOW bit width. To counteract this, a timer element is used as 'watchdog,' which reinitializes the MCU after a preset threshold count of timer states. After this internal reset, the HES MCU again looks for synchronization. So, after the link is resumed, synchronization is again established when the next available 'header' is found. In case of long duration link failure, the MCU is reset many times by this process, but the synchronization is not permanently lost. However, some data are lost during the period of snapped link. Finally, the HES module transmits each modified packet using RS-232 protocol to the desktop PC for serial acquisition and automatic storage in text file.

4.3.3 ECG Transmission Using Standard Telephone

Public telephone systems utilize amplitude modulation techniques for the communication of voice data for circuit switch messaging. Plain old telephone service [originally post office telephone service/system (POTS)] designed for voice-grade telephone service (in a band of 300–3,400 Hz). It is up graded to touch-tone dialing electronics phone exchange and fiber optic communication into PSTN. The rooms within a building and buildings within a complex now-a-days are also networked with the concept of PSTN. Electronic private automatic branch exchange (EPABX) acts as local exchange from where all these rooms are connected (mostly through wires) to constitute the 'intercom' and users of intercom can exchange their words through their private exchange. One or more trunk line from a telephone exchange is redistributed among its users. Thus, a trunk line from the EPABX to Telephone exchange opens up the possibility of networking with rest of the World. A schematic diagram is shown in the Fig. 4.7. The intercom system has been utilized for ECG transmission. The destination number, to which ECG is to be sent to, was dialed first and on getting a 'connected' signal the transmitter started sending the patient ECG data either in real-time mode or 'store and forward' mode. For the latter case, the data is transmitted from its memory where the patient ECG is prestored into the memory of thee embedded module.

In order to make the ECG data receiving automatic, an auto answering machine principle (AMP) was incorporated within the ECG receiver. On getting the ring tone from EPABX for a period of about 3–4 s, the ECG receiver established the connection. The receiver then waits for the required header information in order to start the data recording process if no header appears within a specified time period, it disconnects the line considering it as a wrong call or the call is initiated for talking purposes. It may be mentioned that this ECG receiver line must be a dedicated line.

The basic schematic for the ECG transmission system using standard telephone system is shown in Fig. 4.8. The bi-phase formatted output of the encoder unit MCU was directly connected to the MIC (or speaker) input of the speaker of the telephone set. In the receiver unit, the output was extracted from the earpiece units of the telephone set. For bi-phase encoding, the pulse widths used for encoding bit '0' and '1' were set as 2,500 and 1,250 μs, respectively. Figure 4.9a provides the CRO screen shot for encoded ECG and packet generation from the PES. The output of the receiver is shown in Fig. 4.9b. The decoded bit pattern was sent to the desktop computer using serial port using RS-232 protocol. Details of serial communication between the MCU and MATLAB platform is discussed in detail in the Sect. 3.5.

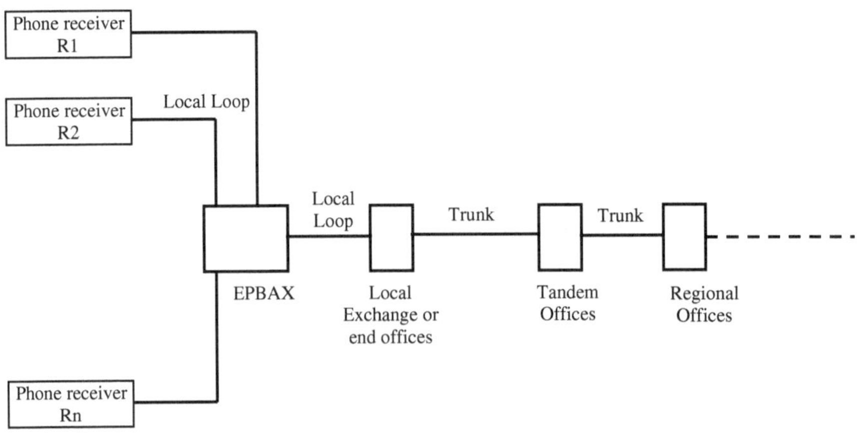

Fig. 4.7 Block schematic of data transfer using PSTN network

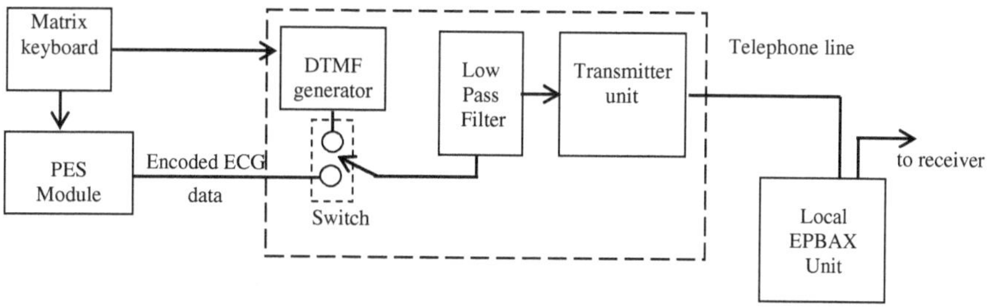

Fig. 4.8 ECG transmission scheme using standard telephone

(a) (b)

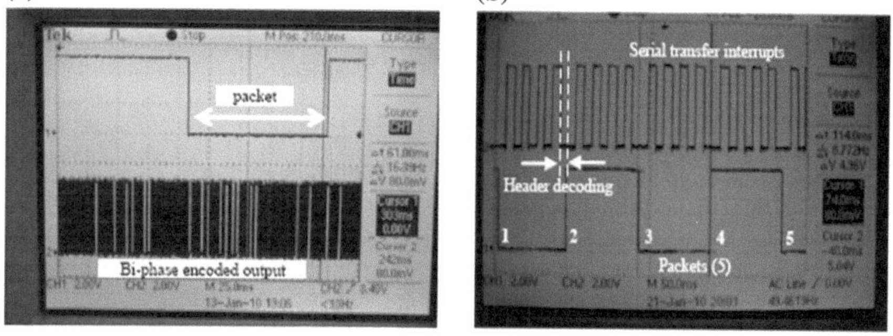

Fig. 4.9 Test results for ECG encoding and detection of header using PSTN communication line. **a** Encoded ECG from PES, **b** Packet detection and serial interrupt generation at receiving end

4.3.4 ECG Transmission Using Wireless Communication

For ECG transmission using wireless communication, Panasonic Make cordless telephone set (model: KX-TG2338BX) operating in 2.4 GHz ISM band was used. Here, the encoded bit stream was DC biased with appropriate value before sending it to the transmitter unit. Since the existing telephone (Cordless) set was utilized for ECG transmission purposes, the primary requirement was to block the DC of the telephone line. Actually in its working, the receiver utilizes DC of the trunk line for its own working supply purposes, the level of which varies from 'On-hook' and 'Off-hook' conditions. The analog receivers modulates this DC trunk line in order to transmit the voice/audio signal (of about 5 kHz bandwidth) using AM or FM principles. Now-a-days digital receivers modulates this line with ASK, FSK, BPSK or even quadrature phase shift key (QPSK) technique in order to achieve all the advantages of digital modulation. The receiver utilized QPSK modulation to transmit the digital bits as well as QPSK demodulation to extract digital bit streams.

(a)

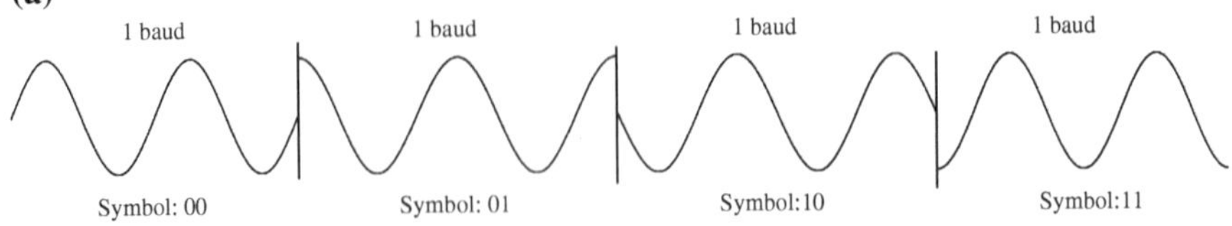

(b)

Dibit	Phase
00	0°
01	90°
10	180°
11	270°

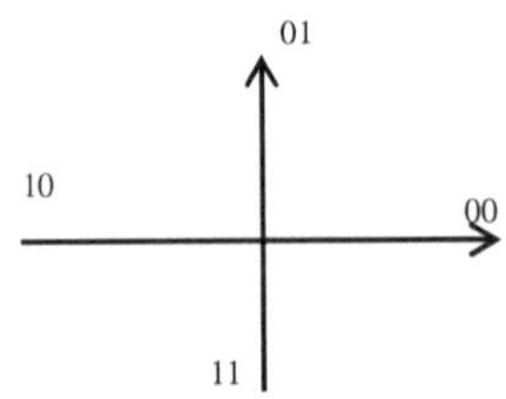

Fig. 4.10 QPSK modulation. **a** Timing diagram, **b** Constellation diagram

Among different phase shift key (PSK) modulation techniques, quadrature PSK has the higher bits per sec communication speed. In general, a bit corresponds to a particular state of the carrier signal in ASK, FSK, OOK, PSK, etc. But in QPSK a state of the carries represents two binary bits which can be realized from the Fig. 4.10a and its corresponding constellation diagram as shown in Fig. 4.10b. Each pair of bits (terms as dibit) corresponds to a particular state of the carrier and it is termed as the symbol or signature. So to represent a byte in QPSK, 4-symbol or signature is required. The details of QPSK modulation can be found at [30, 31].

The purpose of utilizing QPSK modulation is to transmit the dibit symbols over the entire band of telephone line at half of the bits per sec (bps) speed. Generally, the telephone line bandwidths for the voice and data communication are 300–3,300 and 600–3,000 Hz, respectively, as shown in the Fig. 4.11.

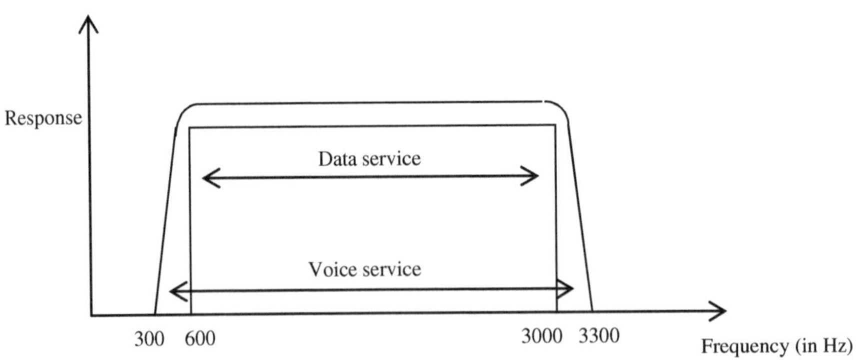

Fig. 4.11 Telephone line data bandwidths for voice and data service

The half-speed transmission of symbols or signatures or bands has many inherent advantages of the communication system, the most effective one of which is to reduce the inter-symbol interference (ISI) due to multipart propagation effect in wireless applications. The overall signal-to-noise ratio is better in reduced speed of communication. The reduced speed also consumes less transmitting power, thus increasing the power spectral density.

In general, telephone application, the voice (analog) signal from microphone is digitized and fed to the QPSK modulation for its transmission. In the developed prototype, ECG signal is not directly fed to the digitizer unit because of the DC like nature of some part of ECG signal. Instead, ECG is digitized first and this digital bit stream is modulated using bi-phase modulation scheme in order to reduce the long-percentage of 'zero' or 'one' bits of digital ECG data. This bi-phase signal (as discuss in Sect. 4.3.1) is fed to speaker input of telephone receiver to transmit it using QPSK modulation.

4.3.5 Spread Spectrum Technique

Spreading the transmission over a wide band makes the transmission look like noise to a traditional narrow band receiver. The spread spectrum (SS) uses mathematical functions to diffuse the signal power over a large range of frequencies. The use of this SS technologies is a must for unlicensed ISM band devices which is imposed by Federal Communications Commission (FCC). Thus, when the SS receiver performs the inverse operation, the smeared out signal is reconstructed as a narrowband signal, and at the same time, any narrow band noise is smeared out so the signal shines through clearly. There are three different techniques for spreading the entire 2.4 GHz ISM band, viz., Frequency Hopping (FH), Direct Sequence (DS) and Orthogonal FDM (OFDM).

In FHSS, the system carrier frequency jumps from one channel to another in a random pattern by transmitting a short burst at each channel with a predefined 'dwell' time. In DSSS, the system spread the power output over a wide frequency band using some mathematical formulations. This system requires more sophisticated signal processing than FHSS process. OFDM divides the available band into several sub bands and encodes a portion of the signal across each sub band in parallel.

The transceiver used in the developed experimentation has adopted DSSS technique to exploit the advantages of SS over cordless communication. In case of wireless communication, the bi-phase encoding was customized to suit the transceivers used. Instead of a simple bi-phase modulation, a modified bi-phase modulation technique was implemented with bit widths 300 and 1,200 μs for bit '1' and '0', respectively. Hence, the frequency of bit '1' was put as four times the same for bit '0'. Figure 4.12a, b shows the CRO screenshots for encoded and decoded bit patterns for ECG signal at the encoding frequencies.

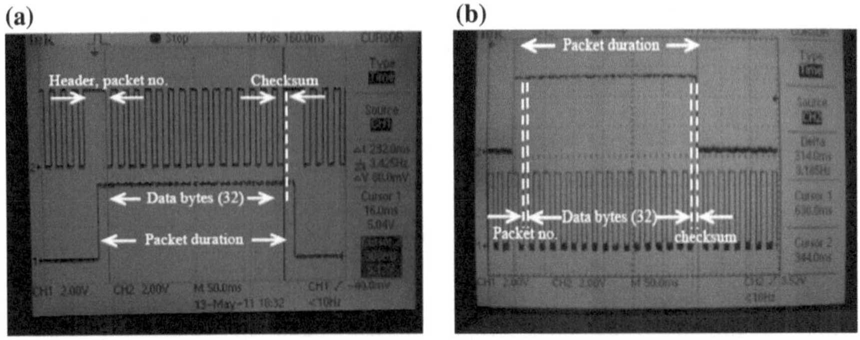

Fig. 4.12 Test results for ECG encoding and detection of header using wireless communication. **a** Encoded packet structure, **b** Decoded packet at the receiving end

4.3.6 Error Correction

Other than the common reasons like multipath propagation, ISI etc., the DC-like nature of the equipotential segments (ST, PQ. and TP) of the ECG signal causes an inherent source of error. This inherent error is beyond the scope of error detection schemes since the transmitted data between these segments are not the exact replica of corresponding portions. Hence, at the receiver end, a distorted ECG will be reproduced.

To avoid this, bi-phase modulation scheme was adopted as described in Sect. 4.3.1. However, data can be corrupted during transmission due to many factors for which one or more bits of a given data units are altered or wiped out. The data link layer of this transmission system was so designed that it is capable to detect any such alteration of one or more bits using the 'checksum' error detection method. The packaging of ECG data, flow control of this packet to the phone set using the available band limited bps selection in the transmitting end belongs to the data link layer. In the receiving end, an addition of decoded data frames from the received bit stream with this flow rate and error correction principle was also adopted. The decoded packets were transferred to the receiving-end desktop PC through serial communication link using RS-232 protocol. The incoming packets are buffered in a temporary file and the BER and PE are computed by the application software using the following formulae:

$$\text{Bit Error Rate (BER)} = \frac{\text{Number of missed bits (or faulty packets)}}{\text{Total number of transmitted bits}} \times 100$$

$$\text{Packet Error (PE)} = \frac{\text{Number of lost packets}}{\text{Total number of packets received}} \times 100 \qquad (4.1)$$

Table 4.1 Coefficient of variation figures

Patient file ID and record number in physionet	Lead	RR duration	QRS interval	QT interval	P-duration	T-duration	QRS amplitude	P amplitude	T amplitude
P237/s0465 (N)	II	1.315	0.174	0.198	0.122	0.186	44.9	2.906	1.655
	aVR	1.588	0.122	0.268	0.636	0.135	11.40	1.005	0.417
	V3	1.502	0.052	0.092	0.177	0.138	2.969	0.039	0.125
	V5	1.444	0.014	0.016	0.221	0.177	3.651	0.221	0.117
P264/s0500 (N)	II	0.386	109	70.01	29.27	1.705	0.162	0.037	0.909
	aVR	0.358	0.185	9.902	116	1.702	59.5	1.987	3.501
	V3	2.127	0.068	0.042	3.758	0.049	1.007	0.016	0.056
	V5	2.247	0	0.024	5.899	0.048	1.075	0.127	0.024
P251/s0506 (N)	II	0.114	0.104	0.278	0.602	0.109	6.491	2.245	0.159
	aVR	0.133	0.150	0.176	0.406	0.138	2.674	11.48	0.656
	V3	1.129	0.061	0.144	0.174	0.086	0.525	0.327	0.164
	V5	1.144	0.018	0.123	0.532	0.091	9.615	0.368	0.198
P276/s0526 (N)	II	0.177	50.10	51	0.513	0.217	32.10	1.476	0.166
	aVR	0.185	42.7	4.012	0.272	0.080	6.852	0.171	0.068
	V3	0.180	0.117	0.147	0.071	0.039	2.029	0.066	0.153
	V5	0.169	0.159	0.184	0.229	1.027	18.02	0.016	0.042
P093/s0375 (MI-Inf)	II	0.886	0.159	14.63	6.340	4.573	8.762	7.196	0.279
	aVR	0.983	0.077	1.149	6.457	1.587	1.871	0.592	16.31
	V3	0.868	0.038	0.052	60.76	0.017	0.038	1.777	0.160
	V5	0.855	0.030	0.031	6.012	0.877	2.084	0.271	0.311

Narration: *N* Normal; *MI* Myocardial Infarction; *Inf* Inferior

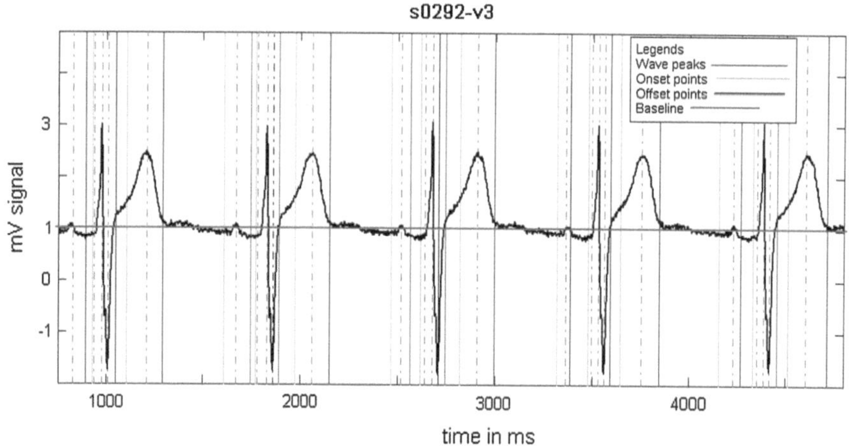

Fig. 4.13 Fiducial points detection from received ECG data

The algorithm steps for computing the BER and PE are given in end of Chapter Appendix 4. If the values are permissible, then the extracted bit streams are extracted and a new file with time-stamped ECG samples was formed.

In the next stage, the application software will compute the wave durations and intervals from the collected ECG data over the wireless link. The processing steps and algorithms are described in Chap. 2. The following ECG time plane features are computed:

(1) RR duration; (2) QRS interval; (3) QT interval; (4) P-wave duration; (5) T-wave duration; (6) QRS amplitude; (7) P-wave amplitude; (8) T-wave amplitude. The extracted wave durations and features are compared with the corresponding ones at the transmit end. Table 4.1 includes the variance figures computed from some of the leads transmitted using the wireless link, computed over 5 beats of ECG data.

Figure 4.13 shows different fiducial points from received data.

A significant improvement in the 'quality of transmission' can be achieved by adopting the principle of 'burst error correction (BEC)'. In BEC principle, 'error correction by retransmission' is adopted where the transmitter waits for automatic repeat request (ARQ) signal from the receiver before transmitting the next packet. If no ARQ is received within a predefined 'timeout' period, the next packet is delivered. This 'stop and wait' ARQ technique could be implemented using a modification of the firmware of the PES MCU.

4.4 Conclusion

Tele-ECG is an emerging area if remote healthcare applications. In this chapter, a brief review of ECG transmission techniques for remote-end acquisition and computerized analysis is described. Our experimentation on ECG transmission using a wire and wireless media for short range of communication is illustrated with a few results.

End of Chapter Appendix 1

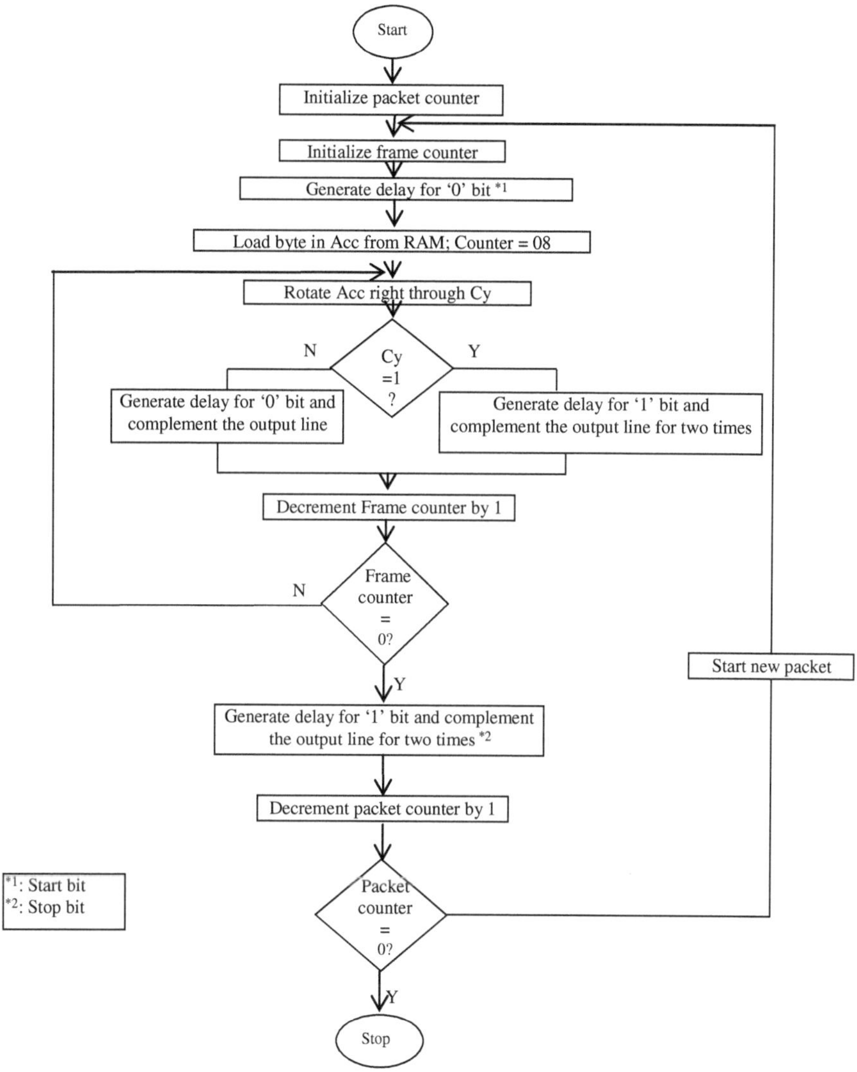

End of Chapter Appendix 2

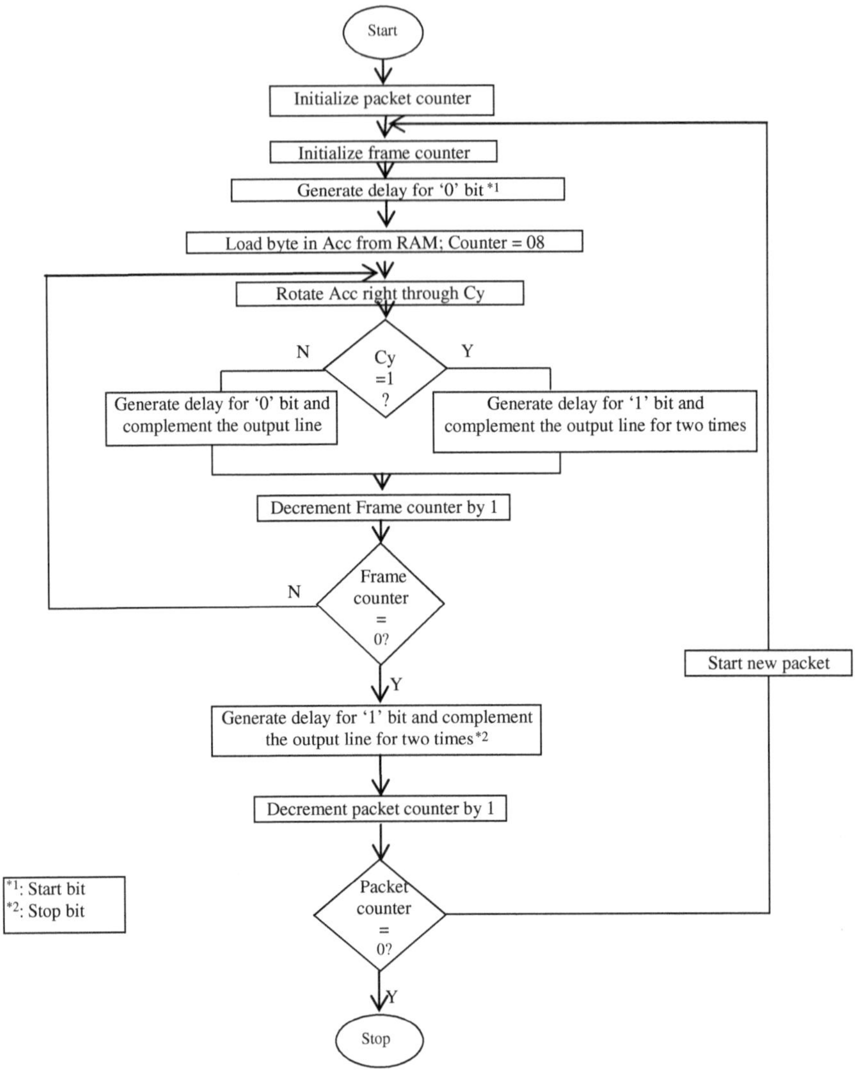

End of Chapter Appendix 3

The algorithm sequence for generating a complete transmitted packet is given below:

k=1; % packet number

cksm = 0 % checksum byte

data pointer = first RAM address

1. j=1; % byte counter
2. send header /'sync pattern' in encoded form with a 10 bit frame
3. cksm = header + cksm
4. send k in encoded form with a 10 bit frame
5. cksm = cksm + k
6. fetch data byte from RAM,
7. increment data pointer
8. send byte in encoded form with a ten bit frame
9. cksm = cksm+ byte
10. j= j + 1
11. if j = 32 go to step 13
12. Go to step 6
13. chk_sm = 2's complement of cksm
14. send chk_sm in encoded form with a 10- bit frame
15. cksm = 0; k = k+1
16. if k= 200 go to step 18
17. go to step 1 for next packet
18. stop

End of Chapter Appendix 4

The algorithm steps for BER and PE estimation is given below:

i = byte number in temporary data file (source);

j = byte number in final data file (destination);

k = bit error index;

p = packet index;

k1 = missed packet index;

x = originating array in temporary data file

y = generated array in final data file;

n = packet number array;

i = 1; p =1; j = 1

1. if x(i) = 'sync word', skip step 2
2. i= i+1 ; go to step1
3. i = i + 1;
4. n(p) = x(i)
5. if p = 1 go to step 8
6. if n(p) – n(p-1)   1go to step 8
7. k1 = k1 + 1;   % missed packets counter
8. i= i + 1;
9. y(j) = x(i)
10. if j = 32; go to step 13
11. i= i + 1; j = j + 1;
12. go to step 9
13. i= i + 1; j= j + 1
14. if x(i) = 0, go to step 16
15. k = k + 1;   % byte error
16. p= p + 1;
17. Packet complete, go to step 1 for next packet

References

1. Watts RP. Some design considerations for narrow-band medical telemetry over the switched-message network. IEEE Trans Commun Technol. 1971;19(3):246–255.
2. Watts MP, Macfarlane PW. 3-lead electrocardiogram transmission over post office telephone lines. Med Biol Eng Compu. 1977;15(3):311–8.
3. Bertrand M, Guardo R, Roberge FA, Blondeau P. Microprocessor application for numerical ECG encoding and transmission. IEEE Proc. 1977;65(5):714–22.
4. Tompkins WJ. Evolution of microcomputer-based medical instrumentation. In: IEEE Proceedings. 1990. pp. 13–15.
5. Guler NF, Fidan U. Wireless transmission of ECG signals. J Med Syst. 2006;30(3):231–5.
6. Patil GM, Subbarao K, Mytri VD, Rajkumar AD, Reddy DN, Satyanarayana K. Embedded microcontroller based digital telemonitoring system for ECG. J Instrum Soc India. 2007;37(2):134–49.
7. Engin M, Caglav E, Engin EZ. Real-time ECG signal transmission via telephone network. Measurement. 2005;37(2):167–71.
8. Oweis RJ, Barhoum A. PIC microcontroller based RF wireless ECG monitoring system. J Med Eng Technol. 2007;31(6):410–8.
9. Bansal D, Khan M, Salhan AK. A computer based wireless system for online acquisition, monitoring and digital processing of ECG waveforms. Comput Biol Med. 2009;39(4):361–7.
10. Lambrew CT, Schuchman WL, Cannon TH. Emergency medical transport systems: use of ECG telemetry. Chest. 1973;63(4):477–82.
11. Pojen MW, Fried DD, Smith S, Lindsay LV, Voigt GC. Studies of ambulance patients with ischemic heart disease. Am J Publ Health. 1977;67(6):527–31.
12. Grim P, Feldman T, Martin M, Donovan R, Nevins V, Childers RW. Cellular telephone transmission of 12-leadelectrocardiograms from ambulance to hospital. Am J Cardiol. 1987;60(8):715–20.
13. Murakami H, Scimizu K, Yamamoto K, Mikami T, Kondo K. Telemedicine using mobile satellite communication. IEEE Trans Biomed Eng. 1994;41(5):488–97.
14. Zyweitz C, Mertins V, Trentina E. Digital ECG transmission from ambulance cars with application of the European Standard Communications Protocol SCP-ECG. In: Proceedings of computers in cardiology. Hannover, Germany; 1994. pp. 341–344.
15. Pavlopoulos S, Dembeyiotis S, Konnis G, Koutsouris D. AMBULANCE-mobile unit for healthcare provision. In: Proceedins of IEEE Engineering Medicine Biology. Amsterdam, Netherlands; October 1996.
16. Qiang Z, Mingshi W. A wireless PDA-based electrocardiogram transmission system for telemedicine. In: Proceedings of 27th IEEE EMBS conference. Shnghai, China; 2005. pp. 3807–3809.
17. Pavlopoulos S, Kyriacou E, Berler A, Dembeyiotis S, Koutsouris D. A novel emergency telemedicine system based on wireless communication-AMBULANCE. IEEE Trans Inf Tech Biomed. 2008;2(4):261–7.
18. Lee HS, Park SH, Woo EJ. Remote patient monitoring service through world-wide web. In: Proceedings of IEEE international conference IEEE/EMBS. Chicago, USA; Oct–Nov 2002. pp. 928–930.
19. Perk SH, Park JH, Ryu SH, Jeong T, Lee HH, Yim CH. Real time monitoring of patients on remote sites. Proc 20th Annu Int Conf IEEE EMBS. 1998;20(3):1321–1325.
20. Nam YH, Halm Z, Chee YJ, Park KS. Development of remote diagnosis system integrating digital telemetry for medicine. Proc 20th Annu Intl Conf IEEE EMBS. 1998;20(20):1170–1173.
21. Magrabi F, Lovell NH, Celler BG. A web-based approach for electrocardiogram monitoring in the home. Int J Med Informatics. 1999;54:145–53.
22. Garcia J, Martinez I, Sornmo L, Olmos S, Mur A, Laguna P. Remote processing server for ECG-based clinical diagnosis support. IEEE Trans Inf Tech Biomed. 2002;6(4):277–84.

23. James DA, Rowlands D, Mahnovetski R, Channells J, Cutmore T. Internet based ECG medical information system. Aust Phys Eng Sci Med. 2003;26(1):25–29.
24. Bousseljot R, Grieger U, Kreiseler D, Schmitz L. Internet-based ECG-evaluation and follow-up, 2nd open ECG workshop. Berlin, Germany; April 2004. pp. 53–54.
25. Jasemin Y, Toft E, Nielsen LA. Real time monitoring cardiac patients at distance, 2nd open ECG workshop. Berlin, Germany; April 2004. pp. 48–50.
26. Costa C, Olivera JL. Telecardiology through ubiquitous internet services. Int J Med Inform. 2012;81(9):612–21.
27. Gibson JD, editors. The communications handbook. 2nd ed. USA: CRC Press LLC. 2002.
28. Gupta R, Bera JN, Mitra M. A Bi-phase enabled serial acquisition system for remote processing of digitized ECG. Comput Electr Eng. 2012;38(1):68–74. (The contribution from Biomedical Signal acquisition and Processing research group at Department of Applied Physics, University of Calcutta, India).
29. Gupta R, Bera JN, Mitra M. An intelligent telecardiology system for offline wireless transmission and remote analysis of ECG. J Med Eng Technol (Informa Healthcare). 2012;36(7):358–65. (The contribution from Biomedical Signal acquisition and Processing research group at Department of Applied Physics, University of Calcutta, India).
30. Madhow U. Fundamentals of digital communication. UK: Cambridge University Press; 2008.
31. Farauzan BA. Data communications and networking. 4th ed. New York: Tata McGraw-Hills; 2009.

Chapter 5
ECG Compression

5.1 Introduction

Compression techniques for biomedical data have been an active area of research for the last 50 years or more. There are two principal areas of application of biosignal compression, viz. (a) efficient recording and processing of long duration patient data (typically ECG, PPG, etc.) for off-line evaluation and (b) real-time or off-line transmission of biomedical signals for remote-end diagnosis by experts. Among these two, the second one has been extensively used in diversified areas like healthcare systems, military applications, sports physiology, space research, and many more. Remote ECG monitoring of patients has been a prime area of telehealthcare, and data compression plays a significant role in efficient utilization of the communication channel. Telecardiology, a special form of tele-ECG, involves collection of patient's ECG data, its compression, and transmission (real time or off-line) for remote-end acquisition and analysis by cardiac experts. In medical data compression, an important criterion is to preserve the pathological information in the compressed data so that the decompressed data are clinically acceptable to the expert for diagnostic interpretation. Over the years, researchers have prescribed some statistical parameters or measures, which provide an estimation of the reconstruction quality of the compression–decompression algorithms. In this chapter, some useful ECG compression techniques in practice are reviewed. A new technique, which is an adaptation of delta modulation scheme, is described for single-lead ECG compression. An application of the scheme for compression of ECG data and its transmission in a GSM-based communication system is also described.

R. Gupta et al., *ECG Acquisition and Automated Remote Processing*,
DOI: 10.1007/978-81-322-1557-8_5,

5.2 Review of ECG Compression Techniques

In general, data compression techniques can be classified into two broad categories, viz. lossless and lossy. In lossy compression techniques, some information is 'thrown away.' In lossless compression, the signal can be perfectly reconstructed from the compressed data. Most of the biomedical signals include adequate redundant information within the signal, and hence, popular biosignal compression methods employ lossy techniques. For biomedical signal compression, one of the following techniques is used, viz. time domain or direct data compression methods, transformation techniques, and parameter extraction techniques [1]. In direct compression techniques, processing of raw samples (sometimes after a preprocessing) is applied. Such techniques are popular in real-time applications. In general, transformation techniques involve preprocessing of the samples using a linear transform and then encode the expansion coefficients. During reconstruction, an inverse transform is carried out to get back original data, with some error. In parameter extraction methods, some signatures of the ECG dataset such as extreme locations (R-peak, S-peak), zero crossing points, or average slope in individual peaks are computed and stored. Reconstruction is carried out by using appropriate interpolation schemes.

The performance indices used by researchers for describing compression performances and error estimates in the reconstruction are available in the literature. Most common parameters are compression ratio (CR), percentage root mean squared difference (PRD), PRD normalized (PRDN), maximum absolute error (MAE), root mean square error (RMS), signal to noise ratio (SNR), etc. They are defined as follows:

$$\mathrm{CR} = \frac{\text{Input (raw) data file size}}{\text{output (compressed) file data size}} \tag{5.1}$$

$$PRD = 100 \times \sqrt{\frac{\sum_{n=1}^{N} \left(x[n] - \widehat{x}[n]\right)^2}{\sum_{n=1}^{N} (x[n])^2}} \tag{5.2}$$

$$PRDN = 100 \times \sqrt{\frac{\sum_{n=1}^{N} \left(x[n] - \widehat{x}[n]\right)^2}{\sum_{n=1}^{N} (x[n] - \bar{x})^2}} \tag{5.3}$$

$$\mathrm{E}_{\max} = \max\left(x[n] - \widehat{x}[n]\right) \tag{5.4}$$

$$\text{rms} = \sqrt{\frac{\sum_{n=1}^{N} \left[x(n) - \widehat{x}(n)\right]^2}{N}} \tag{5.5}$$

$$\text{SNR} = 10 \log \left[\frac{\sum_{n=1}^{N} [x(n) - \bar{x}]^2}{\sum_{n=1}^{N} \left[x(n) - \widehat{x}(n)\right]^2} \right] \tag{5.6}$$

where

N total number of samples in the dataset;
x[n] actual value of sample n;
$\widehat{x}$[n] corresponding reconstructed value.

'Max' operator extracts maximum element of sample to sample difference array.

A combined performance index indicating compression and PRD together, called quality score (QS) is used, defined as:

$$\text{QS} = \frac{\text{CR}}{\text{PRD}} \tag{5.7}$$

The direct compression schemes utilize amount of redundancies among a group of neighboring ECG samples and operate on inter-sample correlation. Reconstruction of data is carried out by a linear prediction or interpolation technique. A prediction algorithm uses a priori knowledge of some previous samples, whereas interpolation technique requires the same for previous and succeeding samples. Theoretical background of such compression techniques is provided in [2–5]. In tolerance comparison techniques, a preset or threshold is used around a sample point. Whenever the first difference between the reference sample and the following exceeds this value, a line is generated whose parameters (slope and length) are used to represent intermediate points. Otherwise, the following sample is ignored. The amplitude zonal time epoch coding (AZTEC), fan/scan along polynomial approximation (SAPA), turning point (TP), coordinate reduction time encoding system (CORTES) algorithms for ECG compression rely on some principle of tolerance comparison method. AZTEC, developed for real-time ECG compression, is suitable for QRS detection. The ECG data are converted into slope and plateaus, considering three consecutive samples at a time. A CR of 10:1 is reported in [6]. However, the reconstructed data show steplike quantization, which is not suitable for visual analysis by a cardiologist. Few modified AZTEC encoding principle is described in [7, 8]. The TP algorithm utilizes an adaptive down-sampling, where half of the samples are discarded depending on relative slope magnitudes between three consecutive samples of original data. Thus, a CR of 2:1 is straightway achieved without any further coding [9]. CORTES scheme is a real-time combination of TP and AZTEC, which are applied in parallel to ECG samples. TP reveals clinically significant QRS regions, and AZTEC compresses isoelectric regions. The data reconstruction is produced by expanding the AZTEC plateaus, smoothing them, and interpolating between each pair of TP data [10]. A CR of 4.8 and PRD of 7 are reported to be achieved in [11] using CORTES. The fan algorithm [12, 13] was developed for ECG signal transmission. This technique uses a minimum slope principle between two samples to include all intermediate points in the 'coverage angle.' The intermediate points are considered as redundant within this coverage angle. The reconstruction is achieved by expanding the line into discrete points by interpolation. SAPA-2 algorithm includes an additional slope in addition to two lines representing the coverage angle described in fan. DPCM is perhaps the simplest compression technique where the first difference of the samples is encoded. The compression based on this scheme is called 'delta coding' [14]. For enhancing the CR, a modified delta coding is described in [15] where the differences between successive ECG samples are compared with a threshold and if exceed this threshold, are kept, and otherwise discarded. At 1-kHz sampling of ECG data, this method achieved a CR of 10. An exhaustive discussion and test results with direct data compression techniques and their suitability for telemedicine are available in [16, 17].

Many of the transform domain techniques have been employed for multilead ECG signals. Here, after preprocessing of the signal, a liner orthogonal transform is used to convert the ECG samples from time domain to a different domain. The coefficients generated are then appropriately encoded to compress the data. Popular transform techniques employ either discrete cosine transform (DCT), Karhunen–Loève transform (KLT), or wavelet transform (WT). A DCT-based compression technique is described [18], where a quantization scheme is adopted to approximate the coefficients for reconstruction of the ECG. Three levels of quantization, viz. 1-, 3-, and 4-bit were used with a fixed and variable threshold level separately. A multichannel ECG compression technique is described in [19]. In this work, a preprocessor discards the redundant ECG channels (III, aVR, aVL, and aVF) and the rest of the channels are fed to the liner transformer. The paper compares the compression performance using KLT and DCT. In [20], the authors report orthogonal transforms, Haar and Cosine to achieve a 3:1 compression for ECG signals. WT-based ECG compression has been extensively used by researchers in telecardiology applications for the last decade. In [21], a new approach using orthogonal zonal wavelet packet compression (OZWC) to model a GSM-based mobile telecardiology system is described. Using three different quantization levels, viz. 8, 12, and 16 bits, the authors report CR values of 18.32, 8.16, and 5.45, respectively, and PRD values of 0.5967, 0.5778, and 0.5759, respectively, using record 100 from MIT-BIH arrhythmia data. For reconstruction performance, the authors used different wavelets like Haar, Coiflets, Daubechies, Symlets. In another application for continuous ECG transmission [22], the authors describe a wavelet-based low delay ECG compression algorithm (WLDECG) to reduce the delay associated with frame size in wavelet transformation as much as possible, without causing deterioration in the reconstructed ECG signal quality. The approach divides an ECG beat into two cycles based on standard deviation (SD), viz. complex (QRS regions where SD values are high) and plain (non-QRS regions where SD values are low). For real-time application, the block segmentations are done based on continuous SD computations and comparing with a threshold. Accordingly, bits are allocated in proportion to the respective SD of the identified blocks. The blocks are compressed using bi-orthogonal wavelet filter and coded bit stream generated integer significance coefficients. Header for each type of packet is determined based on some statistical parameter of the block and sizes of coefficients. For evaluation, MIT-BIH arrhythmia database was used. In [23], a wavelet threshold-based compression using uniform scalar zero zone quantizer (USZZQ) and Huffman coding of difference significance map is described. The encoding is implemented in two stages, viz. thresholding of wavelet coefficients to increase the energy packing efficiency, followed by quantization of the significant wavelet coefficients using uniform scalar quantizer. Lifting-based WT is used for ECG compression [24].

In parameter extraction technique [25], the ECG signal is analyzed and some important signatures such as wave peaks are determined. The peak picking compression is based on such technique, where the signal is sampled and the extrema (maxima and minima) and other significant points, slope changes, zero crossing levels are stored, with a view to store the maximum information. These parameters are actually stored in place of the samples. For data reconstruction, appropriate interpolation technique is used. In [26], a technique is discussed which utilizes the second-order difference to detect a large curvature point. The maxima and minima positions are 'picked' and saved. The reconstruction is achieved using spline function. In [27], authors describe a similar approach using B-spline function.

Compression assumes special attention for real-time telecardiology applications. For real-time analysis at the receiving end, the decompression time of ECG data should be optimum for faster diagnosis. Conventional ECG compression approaches require decompression of the received packet at the receiving end and this causes some delay. For critical patients, undergoing continuous monitoring applications handheld gadgets such as mobile phones and i-pads are in use for ECG analysis, classification, and alarm generation. In [28], the authors successfully implement a novel system in continuous monitoring application, where the mobile phone of the patient was used for acquisition, compression, and transmission of packets to the hospital server for further analysis using data mining technique. Thus, the entire computational task was shared between mobile phone and hospital server. The server computes the disease identification task such as attribute selection and expectation-maximization-based clustering [29] from the compressed ECG packets. These cluster ranges are sent back to the patient's mobile which uses a rule-based algorithm to classify the patient's ECG in one category, viz. normal, premature ventricular contraction (PVC), atrial fibrillation, and atrial premature beat (APB). Use of public communication network for real time transmission of patient ECG is common practice in advanced nations. Security of patients' identity is essential [30, 31]. In [32], the authors present an encoding technique which includes ECG compression and encryption. The compression technique adopts an adaptation of delta encoding in a mobile phone platform.

An important criterion for ECG compression is the clinical validity of the reconstructed signal for diagnosis. In [33], some distortion measures based for QRS complex, P and T waves are proposed. These include duration and shape of QRS, P and T waves, their durations, ST segment elevation, etc. In [34], the authors proposed a total of 18 distortion measures in decompressed ECG signal, which included magnitude, slope, and shape of all constituent wave and segments of ECG. A critical discussion on traditional distortion measures (like PRD) has been carried out in [35] which advocates for wavelet-based diagnostic distortion measure to obtain superior results. The same authors proposed a multiscale entropy-based wavelet distortion measures in [36].

5.3 Proposed ECG Compression Scheme

In the following sections, an ECG encoding technique based on direct data compression (DDC) is described. The scheme is developed for off-line compression of single-channel ECG using 8-bit resolution and an adaptation of delta modulation. The technique is computationally simple and found equally suitable for tele-ECG applications as well as archiving of ECG data.

A typical ECG cycles can be divided into two zones, viz. QRS, where fluctuation is high, and non-QRS, where fluctuation is low. Now, if the first difference (also called successive sample difference, or SSD) of the ECG sample is computed and compared with the original ECG plot (Fig. 5.1), it is seen that the fluctuations in the SSD array is confined to almost 15% of the total array, in QRS regions, as indicated by red color as shown in Fig. 5.1.

The fluctuations in the non-QRS zones are either minimum (P and T waves) or almost nil (isoelectric segments), of the order of 10^{-2} in millivolt scale. In the

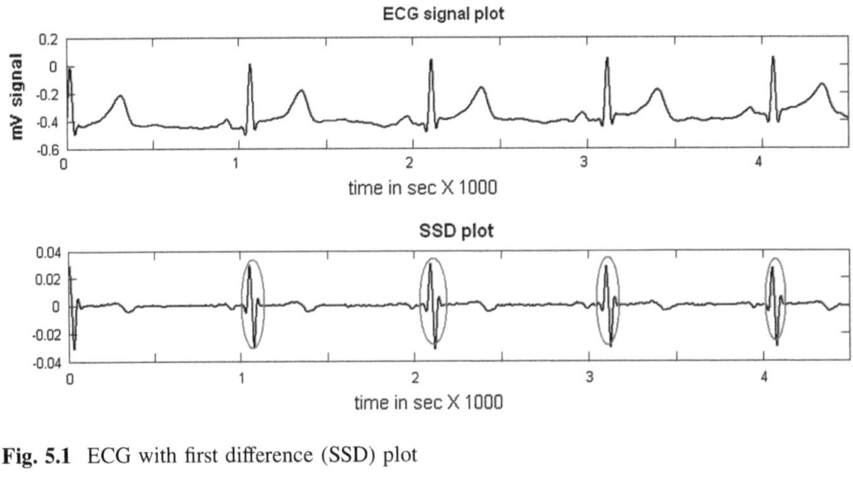

Fig. 5.1 ECG with first difference (SSD) plot

developed compression scheme, encoding is performed using the following two rules:

Rule (A): In P and T wave regions, the first difference elements can be suitably normalized (in a scale of 0–100) and can be represented by a nibble instead of a byte. Hence, in principle, magnitudes of two such consecutive elements can be represented by a single byte. Thus, a direct 2:1 compression is achieved.
Rule (B): In isoelectric regions (TP, ST, and PQ), many consecutive first difference elements, normalized in a scale of 0–100, assume zero values. Each such zero sequence can be represented by a single byte, representing the total number of consecutive zero elements.

5.3.1 Stages of Encoding

Encoding of the single-channel ECG is initiated with a two-column text file containing data samples against the respective sampling instants. Since the sampling interval is uniform, a single byte is used to encode the sampling information which is embedded with the final encoded data stream. Hence, compression stages are applied on millivolt samples only. The stages of compression are described in Fig. 5.2. At first, removal of high-frequency noise from the data samples is done. The first difference array is computed using the following formula:

$$y(i) = x(i+1) - x(i) \tag{5.8}$$

To account for the sign of the first difference array elements, a separate encoding scheme is used. For this, data grouping is done and then Rule (A) followed by Rule (B) is applied in sequence. During the reconstruction (decompression) process, the samples will be generated by cumulative addition of first difference values with the first sample.

Finally, the encoded elements are stored as 8-bit ACSII characters. The following subsections represent the stages of compression.

At first, the raw sample dataset is smoothed depending on the span of the dataset by 'spline' smoothing function to eliminate the high-frequency noise. The smoothing factor is empirically selected as 0.001 fraction of the amplitude span of the raw dataset. The first difference array elements, computed by Eq. 5.8, are normalized using a factor (k) determined in the following manner:

$$k = \frac{99}{\max[\text{abs}(y_{\max})]} \tag{5.9}$$

where $y_{\max}$ is the maximum amplitude value of first difference array.

Now, since the elements near the isoelectric region are having low amplitude, the first element h is selected near the mid-height level of QRS:

$$h \geq \text{abs}(y_{\max})/2 \tag{5.10}$$

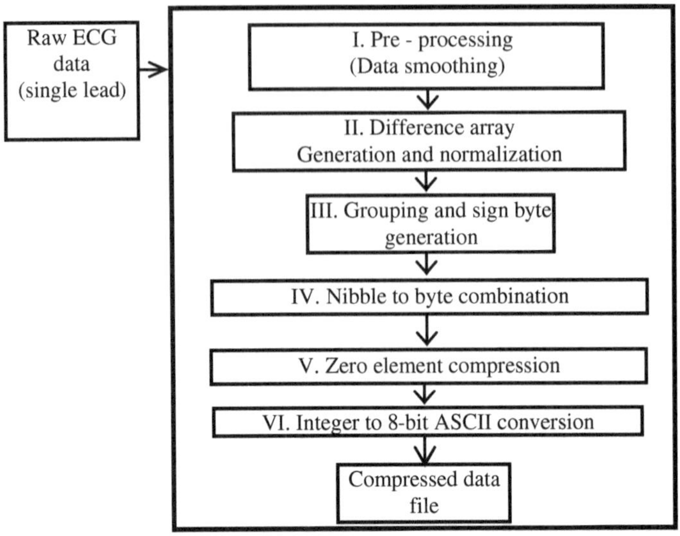

Fig. 5.2 Stages of compression

The elements from the beginning of array y[] up to index h are discarded. The normalized first difference array is formed in a new array b[] in the following way:

$$b(i) = k \times x(i) \quad \text{for} \quad i = 1,\ 1000,\ 2000 \tag{5.11}$$

$$b(i) = \text{round}[k \times y(i)] \quad \text{for} \quad k = 1 - 999, 1001 - 1999 \tag{5.12}$$

where the ‘round’ operator converts to the nearest integer.

This rounding operation results in a quantization error. During the reconstruction process, while the first difference elements are cumulatively added with the first element to generate the original samples, this quantization error can become significant after few thousand samples along the array. To minimize this, the original normalized sample is incorporated after a fixed interval (here, 1,000 first difference elements). Again, the magnitude of elements 1, 1,000, 2,000, etc., may be much greater than 99. So, each of these elements are split into 3 parts, each of which can have maximum value of 99. The splitting is performed as follows: Considering $b(1) = 205.32$ (normalized original sample)

The split bytes b_{11}, b_{12}, and b_{13} from the original byte $b(1)$ are generated as:

$$b_{11} = \text{fix}[b(1)/100] = 02$$
$$b_{12} = \text{fix}[b(1) - b_{11} \times 100] = 05$$
$$b_{13} = \text{fix}[\{b(1) - b_{11} \times 100 - b_{12}\} \times 100] = 32$$

The elements b_{11}, b_{12}, and b_{13} are placed as first three elements c_1, c_2, and c_3 of a new array c[]. The following 999 elements c(4) to c(1002) are the elements b(2) to b(999). So, each block of 1,000 elements from array b generates 1,002 elements in

Split value of b1			elements b2 – b999				Split value of b1000			elements b1001–b1999				split value of b2000				
c1	c2	c 3	c 4			c1002	c1003	c1004	c1005				c2004	c2005	c2006	c2007		

Fig. 5.3 Data grouping illustrated

array c. For next block, element b(1000) will be split and placed as element c(1003), c(1004), and c(1005). Following, b(1001) to b(1999) will be placed as c(1006) to c(2004) and so on as illustrated in Fig. 5.3.

The algorithm steps for generating array c[] from array b[] are provided in End of Chapter Appendix 1.

Since the elements in array c[] may either be positive, negative, or even zero, a suitable sign encoding is now necessary to proceed with further compression stages. This corresponds to steps III and IV in Fig. 5.2. The elements of the generated array c[] are grouped with 8 consecutive elements taken together. The excess elements (n–h) toward the end of the initial array y are padded with zero elements. Magnitude and sign encoding are separately performed for each group of elements, and a new array d[] is generated. Each element in array c[] can be represented as:

$$C_i = S_i.M_i \tag{5.13}$$

where the sign of ith element C_i is represented by S_i, which may be +1 or −1, and Mi represents the absolute value of ith element C_i.

The sign elements can be represented with a matrix as follows:

$$S = \begin{bmatrix} s_1 s_2 \ldots\ldots s_8 \\ s_9 s_{10} \ldots\ldots \\ \ldots\ldots\ldots\ldots \\ s_{n-7} \ldots\ldots s_n \end{bmatrix} \tag{5.14}$$

where each row corresponds to the sign information of corresponding group of 8 elements. In sign encoding scheme, the sign of each element in array c[] is represented by a single bit, with bit ‘0’ (‘1’) representing positive (negative). Thus, a single byte in array d[] can be used to represent combined sign information of corresponding group of 8 elements in array c[]. The encoding rule is:

$$\begin{aligned} \text{if } S_i &= +1 \text{ then encoded bit } d_{8-i} = 0 \\ S_i &= -1 \text{ then encoded bit } d_{8-i} = 1 \end{aligned}$$

For an example, for eight successive elements $c_1\, c_2 \ldots\ldots\, c_8 = 2, 5, 32, 3, -1, -3, 0, 0$, the corresponding sign elements are given as $s_1\, s_2 \ldots.\, s_8 = [1\ 1\ 1\ 1\ -1\ -1\ 1\ 1]$.

So, the sign encoded bits are $[d_7 d_6 \ldots.d_0] = [0\ 0\ 0\ 0\ 1\ 1\ 0\ 0] = (12)_{10.}$

The magnitude encoding (step IV in Fig. 5.2) is performed simultaneously with sign encoding and grouping operation, for each group of 8 elements of array c[]. Since array c[] deals with positive integers, the magnitude encoding is performed by Rule (A), taking two consecutive elements together. If both of them are less than 10, they are nibble combined to form a single encoded byte. So, a combined encoded byte in d[] can have value 0–99. Hence, a 2:1 compression is achieved here. Else, two new encoded elements are generated, each having value same as generating elements, with an offset of 100. In such a case, no compression is achieved. So, uncombined encoded elements can have value 100–199.

The generalized structure of magnitude and sign encoding scheme and generation of array *d* is represented in Fig. 5.4. Hence, the number of magnitude encoded elements in array d[] corresponding to each group in array c[] may be minimum 4 (maximum combinations) to maximum 8 (no combination). So, a group of 8 elements in array c[] is encoded as a single encoded sign byte followed by magnitude encoded elements.

An illustrative example is shown in Fig. 5.5 using first group of 8 elements in array c[]. The encoded sign byte of next group of elements c_9–c_{16} is placed in d_8, and corresponding magnitude encoded elements are to be placed from d_9 onwards, and so on.

The next step utilizes Rule (B) to encode the zero sequences arising out of the isoelectric segments PQ, ST, and TP of the ECG waveform. The first difference array corresponding to these portions, after quantization and rounding off generate a number of consecutive zero elements. A first stage 2:1 compression takes place at the magnitude encoding phase, i.e., during formation of array d[], where two successive zeros are nibble combined to form a single zero element. Even after that, there may be occurrences of consecutive zero elements in array d[], if array c[] contains more than 4 consecutive zero elements. An encoding scheme for zero sequence compression is devised by which a new array e[] is generated. The

d1	d2 . . d6	d7	d8 ...	...
Encoded Sign byte (c1-c8)	Encoded magnitude elements (c1-c8)	Encoded Sign byte (c9-c16)	Encoded magnitude elements (c9-c16)	...

Fig. 5.4 Generalized structure of array d[]

c1	c2	c3	c4	c5	c6	c7	c8	c9	c10	c11	c12	
02	05	32	03	-01	-03	0	0	...	...	...	...	...

Originating array c[] - (c_1-c_8)

d1	d2	d3	d4	d5	d6	d8	d9	d10	d11	d12	....
12	25	132	103	13	0						....
sign	magnitude encoding					sign	magnitude encoding				....

Encoded elements in array d[] - (d_1-d_6)

Fig. 5.5 Illustration of sign and magnitude encoding

non-zero elements of array d[] are copied in new array e[], while each zero sequence is represented by two-byte combination. The first element is fixed as 255. The second element is equal to 200 plus the number of successive zeros.

So, encoding rule for sequence of n-consecutive zeros:

First encoded byte = 255 (fixed)
Second encoded byte = 255 + n, where $n \geq 1$

For example, a sequence of 15 zeros will be encoded as 255 and 215 combination. Now, if the number of zeros exceeds 54, the second element exceeds 255 and hence cannot be represented by a byte. Therefore, the excess number of zeros above 254 will be represented by a separate two-byte combination. For example, a sequence of 59 zero elements will be represented as (255, 254) and (255, 205) combination.

Table 5.1 summarizes the encoding rules described in Sect. 5.3.1.

For proper reconstruction, the amplified sampling time of the original dataset and the normalization constant (k) are essential to be available to the decoding device. Hence, these are prefixed as first five elements of the data array e[]. The decoder extracts these five elements from the encoded byte stream and starts decoding from 6th element onwards. After this final stage of compression, the array elements in e[] are converted to corresponding 8-bit ASCII character and stored sequentially in a data file, which is the final version of compressed data.

5.3.2 *Stages of Decoding*

The decompression algorithm developed follows an exact inverse sequence w.r.t. compression stages to generate the original ECG samples. The starting point of decompression is the ASCII formatted 8-bit data. So, at first, these are converted into corresponding unsigned integer and a new array w[] is formed. The first 5 elements of this array are extracted out, and a new array p[] is formed from 6th element of w[]. The successive stages of decompression are described in following sections.

The decompression process starts with zero element extraction in array p[] by searching a consecutive byte pair 255 followed by a number between 200 and 254. The other elements are just copied in the new array q[]. At first, the number of

Table 5.1 Summary of encoding rules

Encoded element	Interpretation for decoding stage
255 followed by a number in the range 200–254	Zero sequence
Any value in the range 0–255 followed by a number less than 200	Sign byte
Any value in the range 0–99	Combined elements
Any value in the range 100–199	Uncombined elements

consecutive zero elements are found out from the second encoded byte (following 255), and an equal number of zeros are placed in array q[]. The algorithm steps for this operation are provided at the End of Chapter Appendix III.

The array q[] consists of elements, some of which are encoded sign bytes, and others encoded magnitude elements, either in combined or in uncombined form. In this stage, the sign as well as magnitude decoding is performed to generate a new array r[]. The first element is a sign byte and decoded to generate the signs of 8 decoded elements of first group. The algorithm step for magnitude and sign decoding is given at the End of Chapter Appendix IV.

The array r[] can be considered to be consisting of groups, each consisting of 1002 elements. The first three elements of each such group are split values of normalized original sample, followed by 999 normalized first difference elements.

At first, the normalization constant is obtained by combining the 2nd to 5th elements of array w[]. For each group, the first element is (original sample) generated by de-normalizing and combining the first three elements of array r[]. The following 999 elements are de-normalized to generate corresponding original first difference. From the first original element, the consecutive original samples are reconstructed by successive addition of de-normalized SSD elements from index 2, using the algorithm given at the End of Chapter Appendix V.

If it is desired to generate a time-stamped ECG data, the sampling time array is generated by an arithmetic progression series by de-normalizing the first element of the array w[]. Finally, a time-stamped two-column data file is generated, where the reconstructed ECG samples are arranged corresponding to their sampling instants.

5.3.3 Test Results

The encoding–decoding process is tested with MIT-BIH arrhythmia data (mit-db), MIT-BIH compression test data (c-db), and PTB diagnostic ECG database from PhysioNet [32].

A total of 240 different normal and abnormal leads from ptb-db are used. Table 5.2 shows some test results with 240 leads for lead I, lead III, lead aVF, and lead v5 from different ptb-db files. The average PRD obtained in these leads are 0.723, 0.721, 0.701, and 3.62, respectively. Considering all 12 leads, an average CR of 25.11 with a PRD 1.525 is obtained. The algorithm is also tested with 60 s mit-db data files. The mit-db files contain 2-lead ECG samples at 360-Hz sampling. At first, these data are up-sampled to 1 kHz using an interpolation technique. A total of 25 different leads are tested. Table 5.3 summarizes the test results with mit-db data. An average CR of 21.05 and PRD of 3.822 are obtained.

Figure 5.6 represents a qualitative representation of one normal and one abnormal ptd-db lead plotted before compression and after reconstruction. Figure 5.7 shows the lead plot of one mit-db before compression and after reconstruction.

Table 5.2 Compression results with ptb-db data

Patient file ID and record no. in PhysioNet	Lead I			Lead III			Lead aVF			Lead v5		
	CR	PRD	QS	CR	PRD	QS	CR	PRD	QS	CR	PRD	QS
P236/s0463(N)	20.72	0.309	67.05	22.76	0.705	32.28	22.87	1.421	16.09	31.33	2.780	11.26
P270/s0507(MI-Ant-Lat)	18.43	0.666	27.67	20.55	0.876	23.45	20.16	1.014	19.88	18.55	0.324	57.25
P271/s0509 (M)	19.65	0.227	86.56	17.21	0.075	229.4	18.32	0.070	261.7	29.60	4.505	6.570
P277/s0527 (N)	28.65	2.320	12.34	25.72	0.385	66.80	32.19	0.546	58.95	42.54	6.571	6.472
P281/s0537	19.59	0.217	90.27	18.21	0.657	27.71	19.02	0.159	119.6	24.05	1.597	15.06
P282/s0539(MI)	16.15	1.515	10.66	18.76	0.314	59.74	19.01	0.333	57.08	21.56	0.461	51.82

Narration *N* normal; *MI* myocardial infarction; *Ant-Lat* anterio latera; *M* myocarditis

Table 5.3 Compression results with mit-db data

Patient file ID in PhysioNet with lead number	CR	PRD	QS
100-v5	22.68	3.225	7.032
101-v1	17.85	1.685	10.59
102-v2	18.02	0.782	23.04
103-v2	22.68	5.626	4.031
104-v2	21.73	3.601	6.034

To assess the preservation of clinical features in the decompressed data, a new set of clinical signatures, named diagnostic distortion factors (DDF), are introduced [37]. These clinical signatures, listed below, are specified from the ECG wave which is essential to be preserved before compression and after reconstruction. These are as follows:

RR_i RR interval;
QRS_{dur} QRS duration;
QT_{int} QT interval;
P_{dur} P width;
R_{amp} R amplitude;
P_{amp} P amplitude;
T_{amp} T amplitude;
S_{amp} S amplitude

The DDF parameter provides a beat-to-beat variation of the feature being investigated, averaged over all cardiac cycles in the dataset. It is estimated with the following formula:

$$DDF_f = \frac{\sum_{i=1}^{n} f_i - f_r}{n} \times 100 \tag{5.15}$$

where

n Total number of complete beats transmitted
f_i Value of signature before compression
f_r Value of signature after reconstruction

For a number of the ptb-db and mit-db data files, the DDF parameters are estimated by both manually and using separate algorithms. Table 5.4 provides an estimate of these DDF parameters, computed over all beats, over the 90 normal and 10 abnormal leads from ptb-db data.

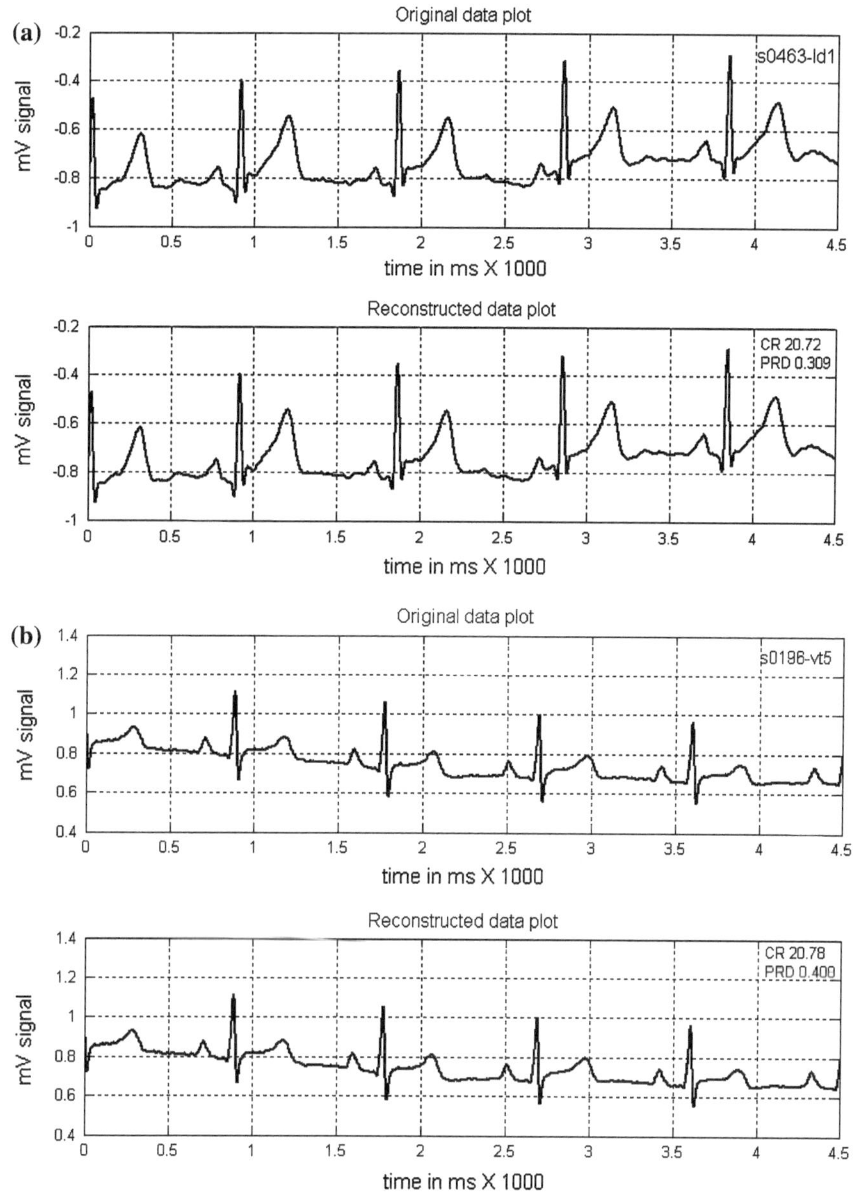

Fig. 5.6 Data plot before compression and after decompression using ptb-db record (**a**) normal data; (**b**) abnormal data

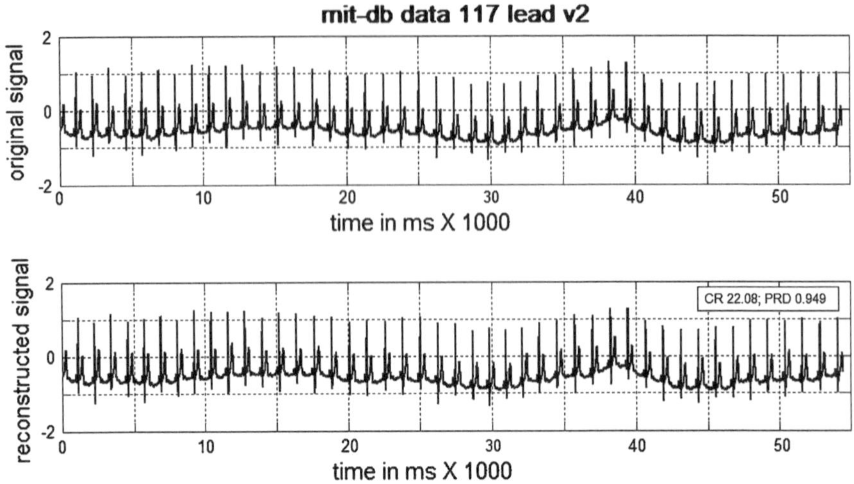

Fig. 5.7 Data plot before compression and after decompression using mit-db record

Table 5.4 DDF parameter estimation for ptb-db (In 10^{-3})

RR_i		QRS_{dur}		QT_{int}		P_{dur}	
Mean	SD	Mean	SD	Mean	SD	Mean	SD
12.3	15.59	32	41.11	22.12	32.1	11.21	47
P_{amp}		S_{amp}		T_{amp}		R_{amp}	
Mean	SD	Mean	SD	Mean	SD	Mean	SD
28.21	25.83	41.38	12.14	5.87	5.21	10.40	9.30

5.3.4 Compression Performance Enhancement by Adaptive Down-Sampling of ECG Array

In the next stage, the effort was to enhance the CR by a down-sampling process of the raw dataset. However, it is also to ensure that the clinical signatures are not affected. To achieve this, the down-sampling is continued and after the first stage (i.e., pre-processing), the extrema (maximum and minimum) of the down-sampled array are checked with the corresponding ones of the original array. Since ECG signal with 1-kHz frequency was used for the validation, 2–3 stages of down-sampling could be achieved using the criteria. For proper reconstruction, the down-sampling factor is to be known to the decoding device, since the reconstructed data need to be generated at 1 kHz. To minimize the quantization error during the normalization procedure, the length of the each packet was (initially, it was 1000, with 1 original sample and 999 first difference elements) also adjusted. Hence, the down-sampling is 'adaptive' in nature.

Table 5.5 PRD and CR values for compression using c–db data

Patient file ID in PhysioNet	Lead 1					Lead 2				
	CR	PRD (%)	PRDN (%)	QS	E_{max}	CR	PRD (%)	PRDN (%)	QS	E_{max}
08730_03	26.97	1.63	1.75	16.54	0.009	25.83	1.66	1.671	15.56	0.014
08730_04	25.33	1.42	1.46	17.83	0.043	25.96	1.31	1.525	19.81	0.019
11950_03	41.12	3.48	7.99	11.81	0.076	39.21	11.98	12.87	3.27	0.117
11247_01	38.11	9.83	9.96	3.87	0.155	33.49	3.42	5.15	9.79	0.040
11247_03	40.16	7.98	8.21	5.03	0.205	40.27	9.73	9.812	4.13	0.030

Table 5.6 PRD and CR values for compression using mit-db data

Patient file ID in PhysioNet with lead no.	CR	PRD (%)	PRDN (%)	QS	Maximum error
101-v1	31.82	1.231	8.359	25.84	0.009
102-v2	32.14	0.435	0.445	73.88	0.043
104-v2	58.64	2.49	2.97	23.55	0.040
105-v1	37.90	2.15	3.228	17.62	0.008

Table 5.5 represents some of the test results with c-db data using this down-sampling technique. An average CR, PRD, PRDN, and E_{max} of 39.12, 4.54, 7.42, and 0.07 are found, respectively.

In the next stage, mit-db data are also used for validating the modified algorithm. Out of 25 individual leads tested, an average CR, PRD, PRDN, QS, and E_{max} obtained are 43.54, 1.73, 3.14, and 0.052, respectively. Table 5.6 shows some of the test results with mit-db data.

Finally, ptb-db data are used for testing the algorithm performance. An average CR and PRD values of 52.04 and 2.12, respectively, are found. Figure 5.8 represents one such c-db and mit-db record being decompressed and compared with original sample.

DDF parameters are also evaluated for estimation of clinical signatures in the reconstructed data. Table 5.7 provides an estimate of DDF parameters before compression and after reconstruction, computed over 2 beats, for 75 mit-db and c-db leads tested using down-sampled data used for compression.

5.3.5 Compression Performance with Thresholding on First-Difference Array

To find the suitability of implementing the compression using 8-bit microcontroller, the PhysioNet data are quantized to 8-bit resolution. Since the PhysioNet data are with 16-bit resolution, to enhance the CR and a threshold value is included while computing the first difference array. Two threshold values 0.39%

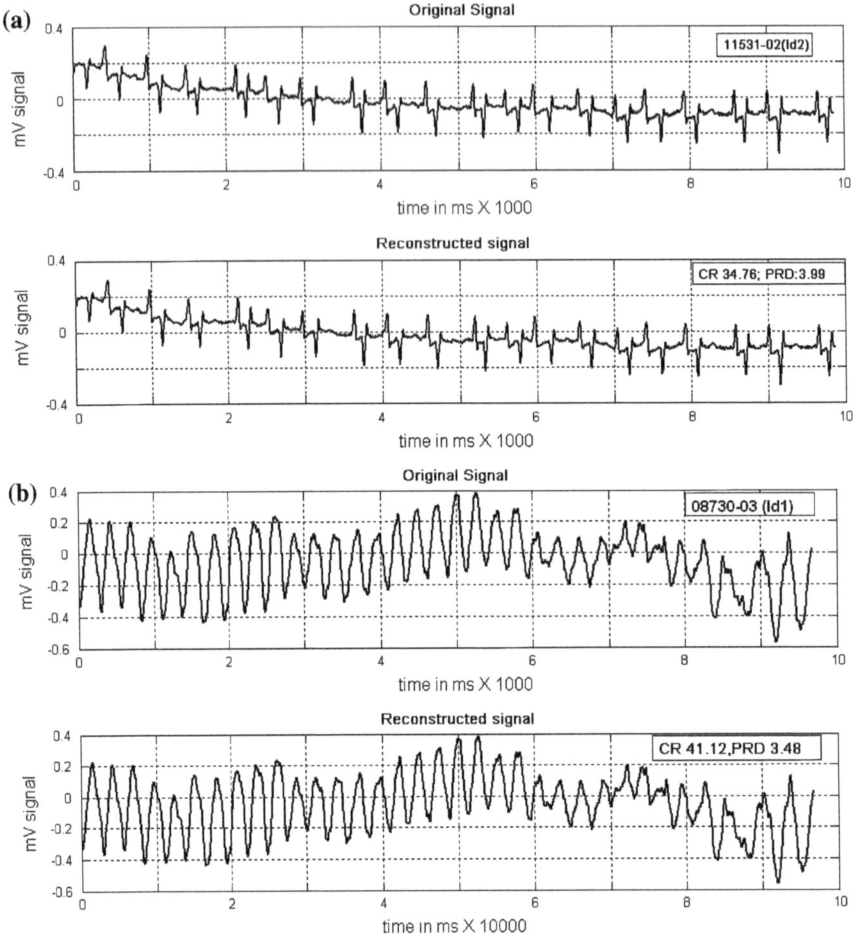

Fig. 5.8 Data plot before compression and after decompression using mit-db record (using down-sampling) (**a**) c-db data; (**b**) mit-db data

Table 5.7 DDF parameter estimation for c–db

RR_i	QRS_{dur}	QT_{int}	P_{width}
0.202	3.72	2.08	1.31
P_{ampl}	S_{ampl}	T_{ampl}	R_{ampl}
0.92	2.2	3.81	1.92

(i.e., 1 in 255) and 0.78 % (i.e., 2 in 255) are used. The differences up to these threshold levels are taken as zero. By this modification, the equipotential segments generate more number of consecutive zero elements, P and T waves are not significantly distorted, and QRS is undistorted. It is observed with threshold of

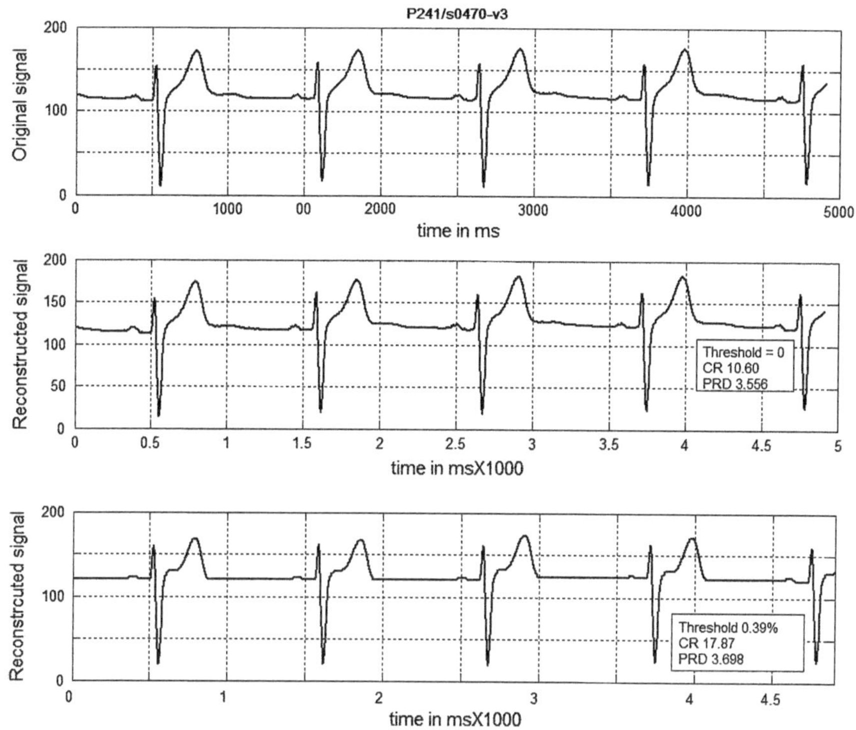

Fig. 5.9 Original and reconstructed quantized signal with different threshold

0.39 %, the CR is doubled in most of the cases with an increase in PRD. Figure 5.9 represents one such ptb-db data reconstructed with and without threshold.

It is observed that the TP and PQ regions have flattened much due to threshold; however, the CR will also increase. Table 5.8 shows the performance of 8-bit quantized ECG compression performance with and without threshold.

However, using a threshold level of 0.78 %, it was found the reconstructed waveform is totally distorted [38].

5.4 GSM Communication for ECG Transmission

In this section, a GSM communication system is illustrated for ECG transmission to a remote mobile phone using the principle illustrated in Sect. 5.3. The objective is to capture a short duration (3–4 beats) ECG, compress the same, and send to a remote cardiologist in the form of short messages to his mobile phone. The received massages can be downloaded to the laptop or desktop for concatenation, decoding and generating the ECG for the cardiologist.

Table 5.8 Compression performance with quantized ECG data from ptb-db

Patient file ID and record no. in PhysioNet		Lead I		Lead III		Lead aVR		Lead v3	
		Th = 0	Th = 1 (0.39 %)	Th = 0	Th = 1 (0.39 %)	Th = 0	Th = 1 (0.39 %)	Th = 0	Th = 1 (0.39 %)
P246/s0478 (N)	PRD	0.158	2.419	4.159	10.46	0.873	15.93	2.695	10.40
	CR	3.31	28.67	4.98	8.86	9.73	33.71	9.60	20.29
P249/s0484 (M)	PRD	0.158	2.419	0.933	8.016	0.085	1.675	1.113	6.095
	CR	5.63	12.20	11.26	35.41	4.48	27.15	15.23	39.15
P010/s0061 (MI-Ant)	PRD	1.504	28.029	0.945	23.90	0.109	2.407	1.901	23.37
	CR	2.98	16.49	3.80	14.89	6.35	37.64	6.46	14.04

Narration N normal; *MI-Ant* myocardial infarction; *M* myocarditis

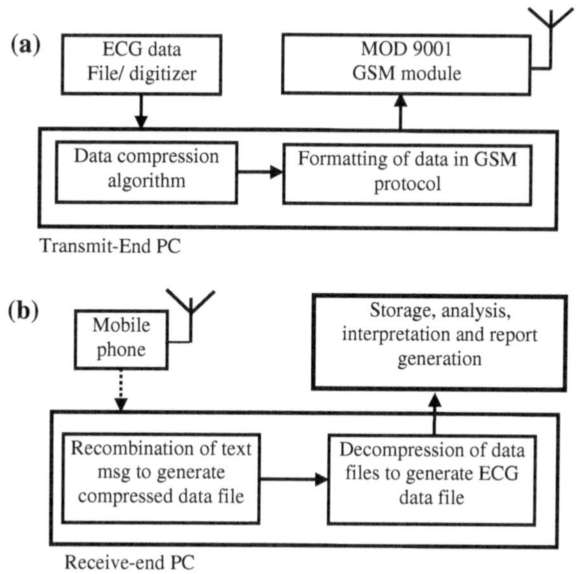

Fig. 5.10 Block diagram of the ECG transmission system in GSM network (**a**) transmit-end configuration; (**b**) receive-end configuration

The schematic block diagram of the developed system is shown in Fig. 5.10. In the transmit end, a PC is used for compression of ECG and transmitting the messages through the GSM modem at the serial port.

5.4.1 Transmit-End Functions

Since mobile message can accommodate 7-bit ASCII characters, the following additional functions are necessary at the transmit end:

(a) Conversion of 8-bit ASCII to 7-bit ASCII.
(b) Data framing for sending the compressed packets through short messages.
(c) Introducing packet serial number for easy concatenation at receive end.

These functions are achieved using a MOD 9001 GSM modem and developing an application software for providing the mobile numbers, ECG file identification for compression, etc.

The algorithm steps for conversion of 8-bit ASCII characters to 7-bit ASCII are provided at the End of Chapter Appendix VI. The protocol frame for sending a single short message through MOD 9001 GSM is shown in Fig. 5.11.

Actual message is prefixed and suffixed by some additional characters, which are directives to the microcontroller of the GSM modem for appropriate actions. The interpretations are given as:

FD	04	10 digit number	Data (7 bit) ASCIII format	0D	0A
Command to send	Target number specifier	Target mobile number	Data packet	End flag	

Fig. 5.11 GSM module protocol

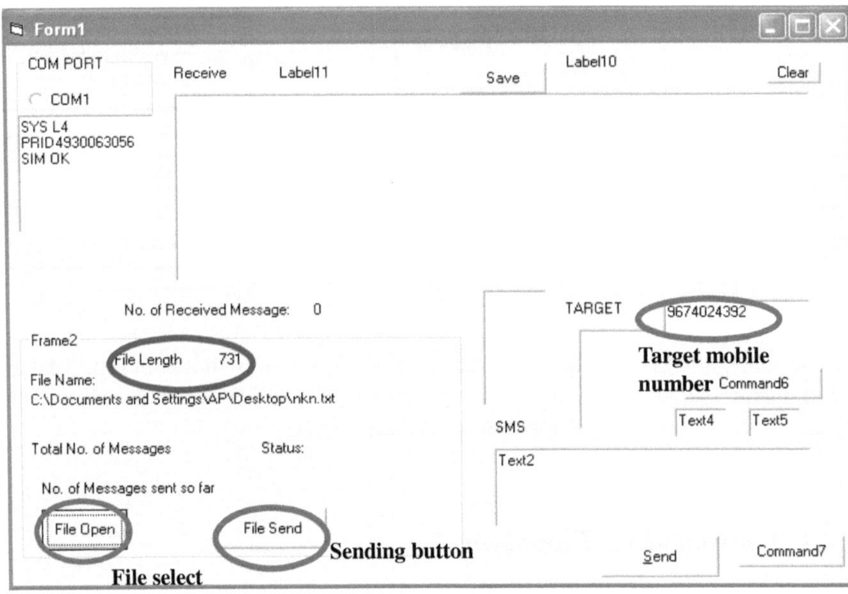

Fig. 5.12 Graphical user interface for transmitting compressed ECG

'command to send': to transmit the message frame.
'target mobile number': 10 digit mobile number of the cardiologist.
'target number specifier': mode of providing the mobile number, i.e., through keyboard, or fixed and embedded within the code, etc.
'end flag': indicating termination of a single message.

Now, a single message can accommodate 160 characters, and an SMS frame can accommodate maximum 80 characters of the original compressed array. A graphical front end is developed to select and upload the compressed data segregated in a number of short messages and deliver each as a frame to the GSM modem through serial port. The GUI is shown in Fig. 5.12.

Fig. 5.13 Sequence of sending short messages

Number of packets	Packet 1	Packet 2	Packet 3	Packet 4
Frame 1	Frame 2	Frame 3	Frame 4	Frame 5

The mobile number of the remote cardiologist is inserted in the GUI front panel directly through keyboard. To account for lost packets (short messages) and their easy concatenation, a message serial number is included at the end (i.e., 160th position) of each data packet (vide Fig. 5.11). The number of total messages can be found out as:

$$\text{Number of messages} = \frac{\text{number of characters in ASCII file} \times 2}{159} + 1 \qquad (5.15)$$

The entire compressed data are transmitted in the sequence as shown in the Fig. 5.13.

The first frame only includes total number of packets being sent. This helps to check whether all message packets are received. The algorithm for sending the data packets through the GSM modem is given in End of Chapter Appendix VII.

5.4.2 Receive-End Functions

The receive-end configuration is shown in Fig. 5.10b. The receive-end application software functions are as follows:

1. Identification and sequencing of the arrived messages based on message serial number.
2. Concatenation of messages by discarding fixed prefixed and suffixed information like senders (Modem's) SIM number, time of generation, receiver's SIM number, etc.
3. Conversion of 7-bit ASCII characters to 8-bit ACII to generate the decoded ECG file,
4. Decompression of the ECG data and generation of graphical plot for visual or software-based analysis.

The cardiologist can send back his comment after his analysis and sending back to the transmit-end PC.

5.5 Conclusion

Compression of medical signals is an essential part of data archival and communication applications. Telecardiology applications require compression of ECG data prior to transmission. This chapter described the different techniques for compression of ECG data. A scheme of direct data compression technique is also described. The technique is applied for compression of ECG data and its transmission via a GSM modem through SMS format.

Note Paper [37] *is the contribution from Biomedical Signal acquisition and Processing research group at Department of Applied Physics, University of Calcutta, India.*

Appendix I

Generation of array c[] from array b[] using data grouping concept

```
t = 0; t2 = 0                          ; initialization
1. c (t+t2+1) = b1(1)                  ; 1st split value of b(t+1)
2. c (t+t2+2) = b2(1)                  ; 2nd split value of b(t+1)
3. c (t+t2+3) = b3(1)                  ; 3rd split value of b(t+1)
4. t1 =2
5. c (t+t2+t1+2) = b(t+t1);
6. t1= t1+1 ;
7. if t+t1<= length of the array b, go to step 11
8. t = t+1000;
9. t2 = t2+2;
10. go to step 1
11. stop
```

Appendix II

The algorithm for magnitude and sign encoding is separately given as follows:

```
% Sign encoding
k = 1;                                   % (source array index)
k1 = 0;                                  % (temporary index)
k2 = 1;                                  % (destination array index)
1. if c(k) > = 0 go to step 4
2. d1(k1) = 1;                           % (encoded sign bit)
3. go to step 5
4. d1(k1) = 0
5. k = k+1; k1 = k1+1;
6. if k1>= 8 skip step 7
7. go to step 1 for next group sign encoding
8. d(k2) = [128*d1(0)) + (64*d1(1))+(32*d1(2))+(16*d1(3))+ (8*d1(4))+(4*d1(5))+(2*d1(6)) + d1(7)];
9. k1 =1; k = k+1; k2 = k2+8;
10. go to step 1 for next sign byte generation
% magnitude encoding (nibble combination)
c: starting array; d: Derived array; d(j) = encoded sign byte,
1. i=1;                                  % (source array index)
2. j= 1;                                 % (destination array index)
3. j= j+1;                               % ( j= 1 place for encoded sign bye)
4. if abs{c(i) }<10 and abs{c(i+1)}< 10 go to step 7
5. d(j)= 100+abs{c(i)}, d(j+1) = 100+abs{c(i+1)};
6. i= i+2; j= j+2; go to step 9
7. d(j)= 10*abs{c(i)} + abs{c(i+1)}
8. j= j+1, i= i+2
9. if i <8 go to step 4
10. group complete, go to step 2 for next group encoding
```

Appendix III

The algorithm steps for zero sequence extraction from encoded (compressed) ECG

p: Source array; q: Derived array

m: total number of elements

i=1; j=1;

1. if p(i) = 255 and p(i+1) >200 go to step 4
2. q(j) = p(i)
3. i = i+1; j = j+1; go to step 7
4. n= p(i+1) - 200 % computing number of successive zero elements
5. put q(j) to q(j+ n) elements = 0
6. i = i+1; j = j+n+1
7. if i < m go to step 1
8. stop

Appendix IV

The algorithm steps for magnitude and sign decoding from encoded (compressed) ECG

q: starting array; r: derived array

i=1; j=1

1. q(i) decode as sign byte
2. i = i+1
3. if q(i) > 100 then go to step 8
4. r(j)= left nibble of q(i)
5. r(j+1)= right nibble of q(i)
6. j= j+2; i= i+1
7. go to step 10
8. r(j) = q(i)-100, r(j+1) = q(i+1)-100
9. j = j+2; i = i+2
10. if j 8 group complete, go to step 1 for next group decoding
11. go to step 3

Appendix V

Generation of original ECG sampled by de-normalization and successive addition:

```
Normalization constant = k;
r = source array;
s = destination array;
i=0;
i1=0;
i2=2;
% generation of the first element of each block of 1000 elements
1. s1(i+1) = (1/100*a)*[r(i+i1+1)*1000+r(i+i1+2)*100+r(i+i1+3)]
2. s(i+1) = s1;
% generation of elements 2-999 of each block
3. s1(i+i2) = r(i+i1+i2+2) / k;
4. s(i+1) = s1(i+i2)+s(i+i2-1);        % successive addition of SSDs
5. i2 = i2+1;
6. if t2 < 1000, go to step 3
7. i = i+1000; i1= i1+2;
8. go to step 1 for next group of 1000 elements
```

Appendix VI

The algorithm steps for 8-bit ASCII to 7-bit ASCII characters.

Appendix VII

Algorithms steps for sending formatted short messages to the GSM module
Serial communication settings for packet delivery MOD9001 GSM modem: Baud 9,600, data bits 8, parity bit none, stop bit 1

1. open the compressed data file
2. put the characters in array x
3. convert characters in x into 7-bit ASCII characters in put in array y.
4. number of SMS to be transmitted, m = (y/159) + 1;
5. get the destination phone number from GUI, and put in variable ph_no
6. form the data packet | transmit header | ph_no | m + 1 | end flag |
7. deliver the packet to GSM modem
8. i = 1; j = 1; msg_sl = 1;
9. if y(i) = $0D_h$ and y(i + 1) = $0A_h$ go to step 13
10. byte_frame (j) = y(i)
11. j = j+1; i = i + 1;
12. go to step 15
13. byte_frame(j) = y(i) + 06; byte_frame(j) = y(i) + 06
14. j = j + 2; i = i+2;
15. if j < 159 go to step 9
16. form the data packet {| transmit header | ph_no, | byte_frame| msg sl no. | end flag |} and deliver to GSM modem using serial port
17. msg_sl = msg_sl + 1;
18. if msg_sl = m go to step 20
19. go to step 9 for next packet formation
20. close the compressed file
21. stop

References

1. Jalaleddine SMS, Hutchens CG, Strattan RD, Coberly WA. ECG data compression techniques: a unified approach. IEEE Trans Biomed Eng. 1990;37(4):329–43.
2. Schafer RW, Rabiner LR. A digital signal processing approach to interpolation. IEEE Proc. 1973;61:692–702.
3. Davisson LD. An approximate theory of prediction for data compression. IEEE Tran Inf Theor. 1967;13(2):274–8.

4. Davisson LD. Data compression using straight line interpolation. IEEE Tran Inf Theor. 1968;14(3):390–4.
5. Kortman CM. Data compression by redundancy reduction. IEEE J Mag. 1967;4(3):133–9.
6. Cox JR, Nolle FM, Fozzard HA, Oliver GC. AZTEC: a preprocessing program for real time ECG rhythm analysis. IEEE Trans Biomed Eng. 1968;15(2):128–9.
7. Kumar V, Saxena SC, Giri VK, Singh D. Improved modified AZTEC technique for ECG data compression: effect of parabolic filter on reconstructed signal. Comput Electri Eng 2005;31(4–5):224–344.
8. Furht B, Perez A. An adaptive real-time ECG compression algorithm with variable threshold. IEEE Trans Biomed Eng. 1988;35(6):489–94.
9. Mueller WC. Arrhythmia detection program for an ambulatory ECG monitor. Biomed Sci Instrum. 1978;14:81–5.
10. Abenstein JP, Tompkins WJ. New data-reduction algorithm for real-time ECG analysis. IEEE Trans Biomed Eng 1982;BME-29(1):43–48.
11. Tompkins WJ, Webster JG, editors. Design of microcomputer based medical instrumentation. NJ, Prentice-Hall: Englewood Cliffs; 1981.
12. Gardenhire LW. ECG compression for biomedical telemetry. In: Caseres CA editors. Biomedical telemetry. New York: Academic; 1965, Chapter 11.
13. Gardenhire LW. Redundancy reduction the key to adaptive telemetry. In: Proceedings 1964 National telemetry conference, 1964. pp. 1–16.
14. Wolf HK, Sherwood J, Rautaharju PM. Digital transmission of electrocardiograms—a new approach. In: Proceedings of 4th Canadian medicine and biology conference, 1972. pp. 39a–39b.
15. Stewart D, Dower GE, Suranyi O. An ECG compression code. Electrocardiology. 1973;6(2):175–6.
16. Kumar V, Saxena SC, Giri VK. Direct data compression of ECG signal for telemedicine. Int J Syst Sci. 2006;37(1):45–63.
17. Kulkarni PK, Kumar V, Verma HK. Direct data compression techniques for ECG signals: effect of sampling frequency on performance. Int J Syst Sci. 1997;28(3):217–28.
18. Allen VA, Belina J. ECG data compression using the discrete cosine transform (DCT). In: Proceedings of computers in cardiology, 11–14 Nov, Durham, NC; 1992. pp. 687–190.
19. Cetin AE, Koymen H, Aydin MC. Multichannel ECG data compression by multirate signal processing and transform domain coding technique. IEEE Trans Biomed Eng. 1993;40(5):495–9.
20. Ahmed N, Milne PJ, Harris SG. Electrocardiographic data compression via orthogonal transforms. IEEE Trans Biomed Eng 1975;BME-22(6):484–487.
21. Istepenian RS, Petrosian A. Optimal zonal wavelet-based ECG data compression for a mobile telecardiology system. IEEE Trans Inf Tech Biomed. 2000;4(3):200–11.
22. Kim BS, Yoo SK, Lee MH. Wavelet-based low-delay ECG compression algorithm for continuous ECG transmission. IEEE Trans Inf Tech Biomed. 2006;10(1):77–83.
23. Manikandan MS, Dandapat S. Wavelet threshold based ECG compression using USZZQ and Huffman coding of DSM. Biomed Signal Process Control. 2006;1(4):261–70.
24. Chan HL, Siao YC, Chen SW, Yu SF. Wavelet based ECG compression by bit-field preserving and running length encoding. Comput Methods Prog Biomed 2008;90(1):1–8.
25. Giakoumakis EA, Papakonstantinou G. An ECG data reduction algorithm. Comput cardiology, Oct 1986, Boston, MA; 1986. pp. 675–677.
26. Imai H, Kiraura N, Yoshida Y. An efficient coding method for electrocardiography using spline function. Syst Comput Jpn. 1985;16(3):85–94.
27. Karczewicz M, Gabbouj M. ECG data compression using spline approximation. Signal Process 1997;59(1):43–59.
28. Sufi F, Kalil I. Diagnosis of cardiovascular abnormalities from compressed ECG: a data mining based approach. IEEE Tran Biomed Eng. 2011;15(1):33–9.
29. Sufi F, Khalil I, Mahmood AN. A clustering based system for instant detection of cardiac abnormalities from compressed ECG. Expert Sys Appl. 2011;38(5):4705–4713.

30. Health Insurance Portability and Accountability Act 1996, 104th Congress, Public law 104–191, 1996.
31. Health Insurance Portability and Accountability Act 1996 (HI-PAA), Centres for Medicine and Medicaid Services, 1996.
32. Sufi F, Kalil I. Enforcing secured ECG transmission for realtime telemonitoring: a joint encoding, compression, encryption mechanism. Secur Comm Netw. 2008;1(5):389–405.
33. Zigel Y, Cohen A, Katz A. A diagnostic meaningful distortion measure for ECG compression. In: Proceedings of 19th convention of electrical and electronics engineers in Israel, Nov 5–6, 1996, Israel; 1996. pp. 117–120.
34. Zigel Y, Cohen A, Katz A. The weighted diagnostic distortion (WDD) measure for ECG signal compression. IEEE Tran Biomed Eng. 2000;47(11):1422–30.
35. Manikandan MS, Dandapat S. ECG distortion measures and their effectiveness. In: Proceedings of 1st international conference on emerging trends in engineering and technology (ICETET '08), July 16–18, 2008, Nagpur, India; 2008. pp. 705–710.
36. Manikandan MS, Dandapat S. Multiscale entropy-based weighted distortion measure for ECG coding. IEEE Signal Process Lett. 2008;15:829–32.
37. Mitra M, Bera JN, Gupta R. Electrocardiogram compression technique for global system of mobile- based offline telecardiology application for rural clinics in India. IET Sci Meas Technol. 2012;6(6):412–9. The contribution from Biomedical Signal acquisition and Processing research group at Department of Applied Physics, University of Calcutta, India.
38. Gupta R, Mitra M. An ECG compression technique for telecardiology application. In: Annual IEEE India conference (INDICON 2011), Dec 16–18, 2011, Hyderabad, India; 2011. pp. 1–4.

Chapter 6
Challenges and Future Trends in Tele-Health services

6.1 Introduction

In the developing nations, the demand for healthcare service is expected to rise in the coming years. Considering the present healthcare infrastructure, remote tele-care will continue to be a dominant mode of delivering healthcare service. Needless to say, technology will play a significant role toward this. The challenge for the medical community, technologists, and service providers will be to deliver the healthcare at affordable cost. The end-users like medical practitioners, para-medics will require more exposure and training toward use of medical equipments and systems. This chapter is aimed to highlight the challenges and trends in tele-health systems.

6.2 Challenges in Remote Healthcare Delivery in Developing Nations

Some of the developing nations have initiated the telemedicine service from 1980s or later. District hospitals have been connected to city-based specialty hospitals by some means of communication network, which may be a broadband connection, satellite link or low-speed PSTN telephone network. Many academic and research institutions have taken up research projects for the development of tele-health services and prototypes have been developed. A wide band of literature is available that tells the success story at the research level. However, in case of developing countries like India, most of the in-service applications are in the project level [1–3]. In [4], a model of the e-health challenges has been discussed in the context of developing nations. The challenges are categorized into: technological and operational, social and cultural, native environment, legal, policymaking and financial. Among these, the technological and operational is the most important and cost-intensive since it contributes to the interfaces of medical equipments, data transfer, and reliability of the medical information to the remote end physician, who can not

R. Gupta et al., *ECG Acquisition and Automated Remote Processing*, DOI: 10.1007/978-81-322-1557-8_6, © Springer India 2014

access (or examine) the patient directly. Information and communication technology plays a significant role in implementing a reliable platform for medical data collection, transmission, and presentation to the physician for remote diagnosis. In many developing countries, since the healthcare sector is primarily government funded, the development of low-cost indigenous technologies can assume vital role. Among the social and cultural challenges, lack of training and mindset toward using computer-based gadgets by the medical community (specially paramedics) is the main hindrance. Awareness build-up among the prime beneficiaries, i.e., patients is also important toward use of new technologies, since a section of people exert disbelief toward new services and technology. Adoption of proper support and legal framework for the usage of electronic equipment, their standards, promotion of e-health in medical education [5], patient data security and usage in research are some of the key issues in the national level health policymaking that can support and expand tele-health services as a whole.

6.3 Zigbee Technology: Use in Healthcare Communication Networks

Zigbee protocol (IEEE 802.15.4) is intended for low power and short to medium distance (within 500 m) communication, with multiple nodes per network. The name comes from Zigzag path of a bee (data packet) between one flower to flower (nodes). Out of the 7-standard open system interface (OSI) communication layers, Zigbee specifies only four layers, viz., Physical (PHY), Data Link (DL), Network (NL) and Application (APL). This helps the system developers to exploit the lower layers to custom their design. Figure 6.1 shows the Zigbee stack. The salient features of Zigbee technology is given in Table 6.1. The IEEE 802.15.4 standard supports multiple layer topologies, including star and peer-to-peer networks, as shown in Fig. 6.2. A Zigbee network uses three devices, viz., network coordinator, full function device and reduced function device. The network coordinator, only one in each network, maintains the overall network knowledge and forms the bridge to other networks. The full function device, also named 'router,' supports all the IEEE 802.15.4 network functions and features specified by the network. It can also function as network coordinator. The reduced function device uses the limited functionality of the Zigbee stack. Detailed information on Zigbee communication can be found in [6–8].

For short-range communication applications in healthcare, viz., patient monitoring, Zigbee technology has already been applied in many countries. In [9], a Zigbee-based outdoor wireless healthcare monitoring system architecture is described. The entire system is divided into two parts: Zigbee-based sensor network platform and host server. The patients are provided with Zigbee-enabled wearable devices which transmit ECG, heart rate, SpO_2, blood pressure (BP), temperature and patient position message to the gateway, which in turn, communicates to the host servers via Ethernet, Wi-Fi or GPRS. In the reported work,

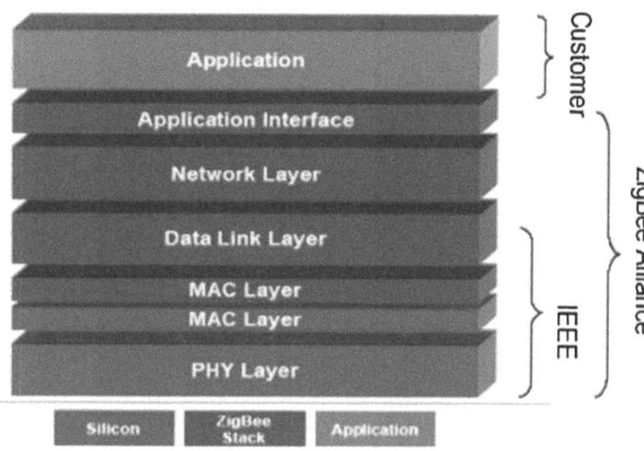

Fig. 6.1 Zigbee stack

Table 6.1 Zigbee at a glance

Features	Specified range
Data rate	(1) 868 MHz: 20 kbps (2) 915 MHz: 40 m kbps (3) 2.4 GHz: 250 kbps
Frequency bands	Physical layers at 868 MHz, 915 MHz and 2.4 GHz
Range of communication	10–1,000 m
Latency	15 ms
Channels	(1) 868/915 MHz: 11 channels (2) 2.4 GHz: 16 channels
Addressing	Short 8 bit or 64 bit IEEE
Channel access	CSMA-CA and slotted CSMA-CA
Temperature range	−40–80 °C

localization accuracy has been increased by utilizing location engine and Manhattan distance localization. In [10], an FPGA-based system, coupled with a Zigbee module is used for wireless monitoring of ECG. The hardware module consists of amplifier, filter, and AD converter and Altera EP2C35 FPGA. The FPGA module transfers the data to the Zigbee module through the serial peripheral interface (SPI) port. The compression in the ECG signal is achieved by linear approximation distance threshold (LIDT) algorithm.

In [11], the authors presented a Zigbee-based any cast routing system for wireless patient monitoring. The system detects patient fall, indoor positioning, and ECG monitoring. When a fall event is detected, the patient module transmits a 4 s. ECG data to the receiver along with patient location information. The authors considered traffic overhead, latencies of the transmitted messages and path recovery, validated by experimental results. The proposed system is useful for the monitoring of elderly patients at hospitals or home. In [12], a wireless single-channel ECG monitor using a TI low-power microcontroller TMS430F149 coupled with a Zigbee module is described. At the patient side, the acquisition module performs the signal conditioning sends the data to the Zigbee through UART link.

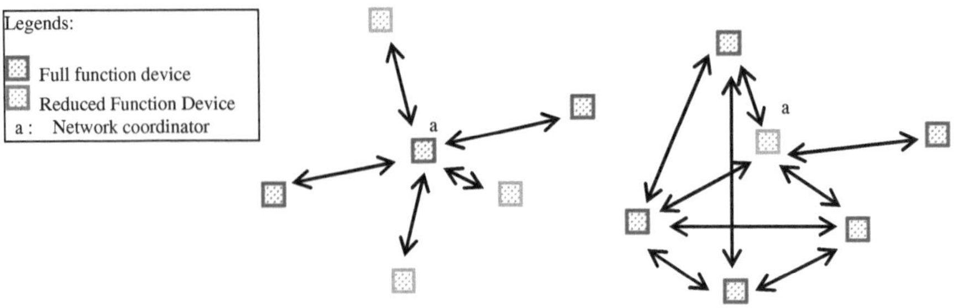

Fig. 6.2 Zigbee network topologies

In the receiving side, Zigbee module delivers the data to the PC through USB. In the host computer, a real-time ECG plot and heart rate measure is provided at the front end. A similar system is reported in [13] where the authors used MSP430FG439 processor coupled with MG2455TAI Zigbee module. In [14], a wireless BP-monitoring system of patients during hemodialysis process is described. The patient end module used TIMSP430F169 microcontroller with XBee 2.4 GHz Zigbee module. The remote end computer generates alarm messages when the BP exceeds normal range. The efficiency of a Zigbee-based ubiquitous healthcare service using mobile phone for elderly patients is investigated in [15]. In this study, blood glucometer and ECG were studied with mobile phone and wireless transmitter, respectively, both enabled with Zigbee protocol. Some recent works on remote health-monitoring applications are given [16–21].

For developing nations, the Zigbee technology can be effective at hospitals for in-house patient monitoring. The only requirement is the proper infrastructure and connectivity with the specialist doctors for clinical advice. Although a lot of research has been done with prototype systems, the patient-monitoring modules, available only from limited vendors in developed nations, are too costly for general usage.

6.4 Requirements for Remote Healthcare Setup

From the discussions in Sect. 1.7 and in the present chapter, development of tele-healthcare in the developing nation requires addressing of some specific issues given below:

Development of nationwide communication infrastructure is the first and foremost criteria. In Indian scenario, the tier-1 cities and most of the districts are well covered by government and/or private service providers' network. However, the remote villages, specially in hill regions, the connectivity and maintenance is still inadequate.

Lack of medical professionals and specialists is a burning issue for most developing nations. To engage or utilize the available specialists for remote health services, they can be provided with gadgets with software for medical data analysis. Most of the city-based doctors use laptops, iPads, or mobile phones. Internet and GPRS can be used for sending the doctors with patients' medical data for their diagnosis and feedback. However, this also requires national-level policy framework for health services. Again, availability of softwares for medical data analysis is an important issue. Presently, these are patented and proprietary items of research laboratories in advanced nations. Here, the government can pay an important role for the distribution of softwares in city-based hospitals and even to the specialist doctors at affordable cost.

The paramedics play an important role in rural healthcare. For the remote healthcare setup in rural clinics, the paramedics are required to be trained for proper use of the communication gadgets, computers, and biomedical equipments.

6.5 Conclusion

In the developing nations, remote healthcare can be effectively used to serve the general population with proper infrastructural facility. In this chapter, the key issues toward implementation of remote healthcare are discussed. The potential of Zigbee technology toward short-range monitoring of patients is explored with some reported work. The main requirements of extending an effective remote healthcare service are also suggested.

References

1. Mishra SK, Basner R, Singh K. Current telemedicine infrastructure, network and applications in India. In: Proceedings of 8th. international conference on e-health networking, applications and services, (HEALTHCOM 2006), Aug 16–19, New Delhi, India; 2006. pp. 46–49.
2. Martinez A, Villarroel V, Seoane J, Pozo FD. Rural telemedicine for primary healthcare in developing countries. IEEE Technol Soc Mag. 2004;23(2):13–22.
3. Trichili H, Dhibi M, Solaiman B. Telemedicine in developing countries: case of Tunisia. In: Proceedings of 3rd. international conference on information and communication technologies: from theory to applications (ICTTA 2008), Apr 7–11, 2004. pp. 1–4.
4. Khalifehsoltani SN, Gerami MR. E-health challenges, opportunities and experiences of developing nations. In: Proceedings of International conference on e-Education, e-business, e-Management and e-Learning, (IC4E'10), Jan 22–24, 2010, Sanya, China; 2010. pp. 264–268.
5. Safwat A, Pouabdolla A. E-learning for healthcare professionals towards HIS in Egypt. In: Proceedings of 7th. international conference on communications and information technology (ICICT), Dec 14–16, 2009, Egypt; 2009. pp. 25–29.
6. Labiod H, Afifi H, Desantis C. WI-FITM, BluetoothTM, ZigbeeTM and WiMAXTM, Springer; 2007.
7. Bandyopadhyay LK, Chaulya SK, Mishra PK. Wireless communication in underground mines RFID based sensor networking, Springer; 2010.
8. Faharani S. Zigbee wireless networks and transceivers. USA: Elsevier; 2008.

9. Xu X, Wu M, Ding C, Sun B, Zhang J. Outdoor wireless healthcare monitoring system for hospital patients based on Zigbee. In proceedings of 5th. IEEE conference on industrial electronics and applications (ICIEA), June 15–17, 2010, Taiwan; 2010. pp. 549–554.
10. Ken C, Xiaoying L. A Zigbee based mesh network for ECG monitoring system. In: 4th international conference on bioinformatics and biomedical engineering (iCBBE), June 18–20, 2010, Guangzhou, China; 2010. pp. 1–4.
11. Chen SK , Kao T, Chan CT , Huang CN, Chiang CY, Lai CY, Tung TH, Wang PC. A reliable transmission protocol for zigbee-base wireless patient monitoring. IEEE Tran Inf Tech Biomed. 2012;16(1):6–16.
12. Auteri V, Roffia L, Lamberti C, Cinotti TS. Zigbee based wireless ECG monitor. In: Proceedings of computers in cardiology, Sept 30 to Oct 3, 2007. pp. 133–137.
13. Yang H, Chai J. A portable wireless ECG monitor based on MSP430FG439. In: Proceedings of international conference on intelligent computation and biomedical instrumentation, December 14–17, 2011, Hubei, China; 2011. pp. 148–151.
14. Du YC, Lee YY, Lu YY, Lin CH, Yu MJ, Chen CL, Chen T. Development of a telecare system based on Zigbee mesh network for monitoring blood pressure of patients with hemodialysis in health care centers. J Med Syst. 2011;35(5):877–883.
15. Lee HK, Lee SH, Ha KS, Jang HC, Chung WY, Kim JY, ChangYS, Yoo DH. Ubiquitous healthcare service using zigbee and mobile phone for elderly patients. Int J Med Inf. 2009;78(3):193–198.
16. Li YZ, Wang L, Wu XM, Zhang YT. Experimental analysis on radio transmission and localization of a Zigbee-based wireless healthcare monitoring platform. In: Proceedings of the 5th international conference on information technology and application in biomedicine, May 30–31, Shenzhen, China; 2008. pp. 488–490.
17. Kim B, Kim Y, Lee I, You I. Design and implementation of a ubiquitous ECG monitoring system using SIP and the zigbee network. In: Proceedings of future generation communication and networking (FGCN 2007), vol 2. Dec 6–8, 2007, Korea; 2007. pp. 599–604.
18. Liu Y, Sahandi R. Zigbee network for remote patient monitoring on general hospital wards. In: Proceedings of 22nd IEEE international symposium on information, communication and automation technologies (ICAT), Oct 29–31, 2009, Bosnia; 2009. pp. 1–7.
19. Lin W. Real time monitoring of electrocardiogram through IEEE802.15.4 network. In: Proceedings of 8th international conference and expo on emerging technologies for a smarter world (CEWIT), Nov 3, 2011, New York; 2011. pp. 1–6.
20. Ken C, Xiaoying L. A zigbee based mesh network for ECG monitoring system. In: Proceedings of 4th international conference on bioinformatics and biomedical engineering (iCBBE), June 18–20, 2010, Chengdu, China; 2010. pp. 1–4.
21. Lee HJ, Kim DO, Kang BJ, Ban SW. Mobile embedded healthcare system working on wireless sensor network. In Proceedings of 3rd international conference on communications and mobile computing (CMC), April 18–20, 2011, China; 2011. pp. 161–164.

Short Profiles of the Authors

Dr. Rajarshi Gupta received his B. Tech, M. Tech, and Ph.D. (Tech) degrees in Instrumentation Engineering from University of Calcutta, India. He is currently an Assistant Professor in Instrumentation Engineering, Department of Applied Physics, University of Calcutta. His research interests include biomedical signal acquisition and telecardiology. He is a recipient of University Gold Medal. He has published 25 research papers in peer-reviewed journals and conferences. He is a member of IEEE, IET (UK), IETE, and BMESI, India.

Dr. Madhuchhanda Mitra has received her B. Tech, M. Tech, and Ph.D. (Tech) degrees in Instrumentation Engineering from University of Calcutta, India. She is currently an Associate Professor and Head, Department of Applied Physics, University of Calcutta. Her research areas include biomedical signal processing, material science, and instrumentation. She has published more than 150 research papers in international journals and conferences. She has coauthored two books, 'Electric Power Quality' from Springer and 'Programmable Logic Controllers and Industrial Automation: An Introduction' from Penram International and four book chapters. She is recipient of University Gold Medal and Griffiths Award from University of Calcutta.

Dr. Jitendranath Bera received his B. Tech and M. Tech degrees in Electrical Engineering from University of Calcutta and Ph.D. (Engg) degree from Jadavpur University, India. He is currently an Associate Professor in Electrical Engineering, Department of Applied Physics, University of Calcutta, India. His research interests include wireless communication and embedded systems, and he has published 50 research papers in peer-reviewed journals and conferences. He is also involved in two government-funded research projects related to wireless communication for remote monitoring of electrical parameters measurement in the department. He is a member of IEEE, IET (UK), and IETE, India.

R. Gupta et al., *ECG Acquisition and Automated Remote Processing*,
DOI: 10.1007/978-81-322-1557-8, © Springer India 2014